The Latino Psychiatric Patient

Assessment and Treatment

The Latino Psychiatric Patient

Assessment and Treatment

Edited by

Alberto G. López, M.D., M.P.H.
Ernestina Carrillo, M.S.W.

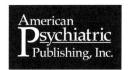

Washington, DC
London, England

Copyright © 2001 American Psychiatric Publishing, Inc.
ALL RIGHTS RESERVED
Manufactured in the United States of America on acid-free paper

04   03   02   01   4   3   2   1
First Edition

American Psychiatric Publishing, Inc.
1400 K Street, NW
Washington, DC 20005
www.appi.org

Library of Congress Cataloging-in-Publication Data
The Latino psychiatric patient : assessment and treatment / edited by Alberto G. López, Ernestina Carrillo. — 1st ed.
>   p. ; cm.
>   Includes bibliographical references and index.
>   ISBN 0-88048-773-9 (alk. paper)
>   1. Hispanic Americans—Mental health. 2. Hispanic Americans—Mental health services. 3. Latin Americans—Mental health. I. López, Alberto G., 1952– . II. Carrillo, Ernestina.
>   [DNLM: 1. Hispanic Americans—psychology. 2. Mental Disorders—ethnology. 3. Cultural Diversity. 4. Psychotherapy—methods. WM 140 L357 2001]
>   RC451.5.H57 L38 2001
>   616.89'0089'68073—dc21

                                                                    00-067625

British Library Cataloguing in Publication Data
A CIP record is available from the British Library.

For my mother, Ana Maria;
my son, Gerardo;
and in loving memory of my brother, Adrian.
(A.G.L.)

With gratitude and love to my parents,
Meregildo and Josephina Carrillo,
and my husband and daughter,
Larry and Eliana Juanita Polon.
(E.C.)

Contents

PART I

Latino Peoples:
Overview and Treatment Issues

PART II

Latino Peoples:
Cultural and Psychiatric Issues

Contributors

Renato D. Alarcón, M.D., M.P.H.
Professor and Vice-Chairman, Department of Psychiatry and Behavioral Sciences, Emory University School of Medicine, Atlanta, Georgia; and Director, Mental Health Service Line, Atlanta VA Medical Center, Atlanta, Georgia

Louis R. Alvarez, M.D., M.P.H.
Director, Dual Diagnosis Program, Arrowhead Regional Medical Center, Colton, California; and Assistant Professor of Psychiatry, Loma Linda University School of Medicine, Loma Linda, California

Heidi M. Bauer, M.D., M.P.H., M.S.
School of Medicine, University of California–San Francisco, San Francisco, California

Jo Ellen Brainin-Rodriguez, M.D.
Associate Clinical Professor, University of California, San Francisco; and Department of Psychiatry, San Francisco General Hospital, San Francisco, California

Glorisa Canino Stolberg, Ph.D.
Professor, Department of Pediatrics, Behavioral Research Center, University of Puerto Rico, Rio Piedras, Puerto Rico

Ian A. Canino, M.D.
Clinical Professor of Psychiatry, College of Physicians and Surgeons, Columbia University, New York, New York

Ernestina Carrillo, M.S.W.
Assistant Clinical Professor, Department of Psychiatry, University of California School of Medicine, San Francisco, California

Carlos B. Cordova, Ed.D.
Professor, Raza Studies Department, College of Ethnic Studies, San Francisco State University, San Francisco, California

Yvette Flores-Ortiz, Ph.D.
Associate Professor, Department of Chicana/Chicano Studies, University of California–Davis, Berkeley, California

Carmen Inoa Vazquez, Ph.D., A.B.P.P.
Clinical Associate Professor, Department of Psychiatry, New York University School of Medicine, New York, New York

Israel Katz, M.D.
Assistant Clinical Professor, Department of Psychiatry, University of California School of Medicine, San Francisco, California

Felix Kury, M.A.
Lecturer, Raza Studies Department, San Francisco State University, San Francisco, California

Alvaro LaCayo, M.D.
Assistant Clinical Professor of Neurology and Psychiatry, University of Florida, School of Medicine, Miami, Florida

Alberto G. López, M.D., M.P.H.
Associate Clinical Professor, University of California School of Medicine, San Francisco, California

Cervando Martinez Jr., M.D.
Professor of Psychiatry and Associate Dean for South Texas Programs and Continuing Medical Education, The University of Texas Health Science Center at San Antonio, San Antonio, Texas

Anna M. Nápoles-Springer, Ph.D.
Research Specialist, Division of General Internal Medicine, Department of Medicine, Medical Effectiveness Research Center for Diverse Populations, University of California–San Francisco, San Francisco, California

Eliseo J. Pérez-Stable, M.D.
Professor of Medicine, Division of General Internal Medicine, Department of Medicine, Medical Effectiveness Research Center for Diverse Populations, University of California–San Francisco, San Francisco, California

Michael A. Rodriguez, M.D., M.P.H.
Assistant Professor (In Residence), Department of Family and Community Medicine, University of California, San Francisco

Ramon A. Rojano, M.D., M.P.H.
Director, City of Hartford Human Services Department, Hartford, Connecticut; Adjunct Faculty of Community Mental Health, University of Connecticut, Hartford, Connecticut

Pedro Ruiz, M.D.
Professor and Vice Chair, Department of Psychiatry and Behavioral Sciences, University of Texas Medical School and Houston Health Science Center, Houston, Texas

Introduction and Acknowledgments

Ms. A is a 52-year-old Afro-Cuban woman with a history of schizoaffective disorder, depressed type. She first received the diagnosis at age 37. Since then, she has had multiple psychiatric hospitalizations, most occurring after she stopped taking her medications. Her symptoms included depression, delusions of persecution, and auditory hallucinations in the form of children's voices. She was assigned to an assertive case management program because she was one of the highest users of psychiatric services in her city.

When Ms. A entered the program, she told her psychiatrist that she did not believe that medication could help with her depression, her delusions of being persecuted, and her auditory hallucinations of voices of children. She believed that another woman, who was jealous of Ms. A's relationship with that woman's husband, had caused her illness. Ms. A believed that she needed a *santero* (Cuban folk healer) to rid her of the jealous woman's evil eye.

In reviewing the patient's previous treatment, the psychiatrist noted that there had been no discussion with the patient about her belief system and about the reason for her medication nonadherence. Nor had there been adequate exploration of the diverse meanings of words in Spanish for Ms. A as compared with someone from another region of Latin America. For example, Ms. A stated that a previous treatment provider had referred her to a *curandero* but that this had not been in agreement with her belief system because "she was from Cuba and not from Mexico." (The *curanderos* of Mexico have different practices from those of the *santeros* of Cuba.)

The case management program set up regular meetings between the patient and a *santero*. The psychiatrist also discussed the importance of psychiatric medication and explained how medication could work in conjunction with the *santero* instead of against him. Ms. A finally agreed to start taking her medication regularly, and she has been out of the psychiatric hospital now for the past 2 years. In the past, she had been able to be out of the hospital for only 6 months at a time.

The case of Ms. A illustrates the importance of understanding cultural factors in the treatment of Latino patients. Ms. A needed treatment that was based on her cultural perception of her illness (going to the folk healer) in addition to more traditional interventions such as medication and case management services. Previous clinicians had not explored the patient's understanding of her illness, and the exploration conducted by the psychiatrist made possible a more empathic connection to the patient and a treatment approach that was more informed and more successful than previous approaches.

The purpose of this book is to help mental health clinicians acquire the knowledge and skills necessary for treating Latino patients in the United States in a culturally sensitive manner that includes an appreciation of the importance of language, culture, religion, gender, sexual orientation, race, and ethnicity in their psychiatric evaluation and care.

The book is divided into three sections:

1. In Part I, we present an overview of Latinos living in the United States, which includes demographic data, statistics on mental and physical health, and a brief history of Latinos in the United States. Elements of a culturally sensitive psychiatric evaluation of Latinos are also discussed in Part I.
2. In Part II, we describe the major Latino subgroups in the United States, along with their characteristics and differences from other Latino subgroups.
3. In Part III, we discuss topics in the treatment of Latinos such as women's issues, substance abuse, and violence in Latino populations.

ACKNOWLEDGMENTS

This book has been inspired by our work with the clients and families who we had the privilege of serving while working as providers on the Latino Psychiatric Treatment Team at San Francisco General Hospital. From them we learned how resilient the human spirit is and how hope and faith can be restored if reached out to with caring and understanding. Throughout the years we were fortunate to work with a team of providers that continuously demonstrated their commitment to our patients by performing on a daily basis those inexplicable acts of kindness that went beyond the call of duty—José Sanchez, Raul Reyes, Eva Del Campo, Alfredo Abarca, Valerie Smith, Johnny Chavez, Olivia Flores, Ellie Dwyer, and the woman who kept us all in line, Angela Barrientos. Unfortunately, there is not room to mention all the staff and trainees who we worked alongside for so long, but from each of them we learned so much. We also want to thank the San Francisco General Hospital Latino Task Force and the Latino Research Program for providing guidance in helping us to conceptualize the ideas that became the proposal for this book.

We have always been fortunate to work collaboratively with community-based treatment providers who also dedicate themselves to the care of Latino clients and their families. We want to acknowledge the work done by the clinicians at Mission Mental Health, El Instituto Familiar de la Raza, La Posada, and La Amistad. Also, our appreciation goes to Tato Torres, who pioneered the development of services for refugees and who has always been a personal support for the both of us.

We want to thank Ricardo Muñoz, Frances Lu, Jo Ann Wile, and Evelyn Lee, who had the vision of developing the Ethnic/Minority Treatment Teams in the Department of Psychiatry at San Francisco General Hospital. Along with being committed to providing linguistic and cultural services to patients, they were also committed to forming ethnic/minority professionals who would provide this care.

We particularly want to express our gratitude to the contributors who made this book possible. We are privileged to have had the honor of working with a group of distinguished scholars and clinicians who have been at the forefront of developing the field of Latino mental health.

We want to thank the staff at the American Psychiatric Press who saw the potential of our ideas and helped us to develop a book proposal—Dr. Carol Nadelson, who encouraged the project; and Claire Reinburg and Elizabeth Gould Leger, who have served as our editors.

We want to thank Sonia Galvez, Jim Barnette, Michael Roach, and Charles Yeh for their assistance with the manuscript preparation, and the staff at our current work sites, Mission Mental Health and the San Francisco Mental Health Rehabilitation Facility, for giving us the opportunity to continue to grow and develop.

I, Alberto, wish to thank my mother, Ana Maria López Elizondo, who sacrificed so much so that I could meet my life goals, and my son, Gerardo, who has made the struggles worthwhile. I also want to acknowledge Dr. Cervanto Martinez, the first Mexican American psychiatrist, for being an outstanding role model and mentor to me and many others.

I, Ernestina, wish to thank my parents, Meregildo and Josephina Carrillo, for giving me the opportunities that have helped me achieve my dreams. I want to thank my sisters, Eliza and Esther, for always being there for me whenever I have needed them. I want to acknowledge my mother-in-law, Edith Polon, whose life story has helped me redefine the meaning of courage. I thank my husband, Larry, and daughter, Eliana Juanita, for giving my life meaning.

Alberto G. López, M.D., M.P.H.

Ernestina Carrillo, M.S.W.

PART I

Latino Peoples:
Overview and Treatment Issues

CHAPTER 1

An Introduction to Latinos in the United States

Alberto G. López, M.D., M.P.H.

Israel Katz, M.D.

AN APPRECIATION OF HISPANICS as a whole is important for understanding individual Latino patients better. In this chapter, we provide an introduction to the demographics, mental health studies, and brief history of Latinos in the United States.

Hispanics in the United States are a large and diverse population. *Hispanics* are defined as individuals living in the United States who trace their cultural heritage to Spanish-speaking countries in Latin America and the Caribbean, to Spain or Mexico, or to Spanish-speaking peoples of the southwestern United States (Valdivieso and Davis 1988). The U.S. Bureau of the Census derived its 1990 data from questionnaires in which Hispanics were defined as persons of Mexican, Puerto Rican, Cuban, or other Spanish/Hispanic origin. "Origin can be viewed as the ancestry, nationality group, lineage, or country of birth of the person or the person's parents or ancestors before their arrival in the United States. Persons of Hispanic origin may be of any race" (U.S. Bureau of the Census 1993).

Although Hispanics may be defined as a population, for the purposes of understanding a Hispanic person and her or his problems, it is useful to see each person along multiple axes or variables. These axes include

- Language (English, Spanish, bilingual, national and indigenous dialects, combinations of English and Spanish)
- Religion (Catholic, Protestant, indigenous, other)
- Geographical origin (North, Central, or South America; the Caribbean; rural; urban; other)
- Class (upper, upper middle, middle, lower middle, poor)
- Race (indigenous, European, African, Asian, other)
- Degree of acculturation
- Gender
- Education
- Sexual orientation

For example, a third-generation Mexican American professional heterosexual woman who has lived all of her life in the United States and who does not speak Spanish is very different from a gay recent immigrant from El Salvador to the United States who does not have a job and who speaks Spanish all the time.

Most Hispanics in the United States were born in, or are descendants of people from, Mexico, Cuba, and Puerto Rico; the great majority of Hispanics in the United States are Mexicans and Mexican Americans. Also in the United States are Central Americans (from countries such as El Salvador, Nicaragua, and Panama) and some South Americans (from countries such as Colombia, Peru, and Argentina). The Central and South Americans are an emerging group within the Hispanic population of the United States. Persons born in Brazil and in places such as Aruba and Guyana are excluded from the discussion of Hispanics in this book because their original inhabitants speak other languages (Dutch, Portuguese) and because their traditions differ somewhat from those of the rest of Latin America. Some other Latin American countries are not addressed in this book because of space limitations or because of the relatively small numbers of their inhabitants living in the United States.

The different groups of Hispanics have their own cuisine, music, literature, dialects, and traditions. Many of these differences may exist even within the same country of origin. This phenomenon also may be seen in the United States. For example, a person from Chicago, Illinois, and someone from rural Alabama are both from the same country but may have marked cultural differences.

Some social scientists have proposed replacing the label *Hispanic* with that of *Latino* (Hayes-Bautista and Chapa 1987; Pérez-Stable 1987), arguing that the label *Latino* better reflects the composition of this population. The terms *Hispanic* and *Latino* are used interchangeably in this book. Table 1–1 describes terms commonly used in the United States when working with the Hispanic population.

Table 1–1. Terms used to describe Hispanics

Latino and *Hispanic*	Refers to persons of Mexican, Puerto Rican, Cuban, or other Latin American descent or origin
Hispano	In the southwestern United States, refers to a descendant of the seventeenth- and eighteenth-century Spanish colonizers
Chicano	Emphasizes cultural, social, and historical ties with Mexican ethnic nationalism and activism
Mexicano	A Mexican person; also sometimes used to refer to Mexican Americans
La raza	A collective term used to describe Spanish-speaking peoples of the Western Hemisphere with a common spirit and heritage

It is important to remember that many Hispanics are not counted as part of the statistics compiled by the U.S. Bureau of the Census because of under-reporting from Hispanic populations. Therefore, the statistics presented may be lower than the actual number of Hispanics in the United States.

DEMOGRAPHICS

According to the 2000 U.S. Census, there were 281.4 million people in the United States, and 35.3 million of these, or about 12.5%, were of Hispanic origin (U.S. Bureau of the Census 2000). The number of Hispanics in the United States grew by almost 13 million people between 1990 and 2000, and the percentage difference for the total population between 1990 and 2000 was 13.2, while the percentage difference for Hispanics was 57.9 during that same period (U.S. Bureau of the Census 2000). The large numbers of immigrants from Central and South American countries, the prevalence of a high birthrate among some Hispanic subgroups, and the relative youth of the Hispanic population are factors that contribute to its large rate of growth in the United States. By 2010, Hispanics may be the second largest racial/ethnic group in the United States (after non-Hispanic whites) (Day 1996). In fact, Los Angeles, California, is now the second-largest Hispanic city in the Americas (after Mexico City).

According to the March 1999 Current Population Survey of the U.S. Bureau of the Census, most Hispanics living in the United States were of Mexican origin (65.2% of all Hispanics), followed by Central and South Americans (14.3%), Puerto Ricans (9.6%), Cubans (4.3%), and other Hispanics (6.6%) (Ramírez 2000). Most Mexican Americans live in the Southwest, especially in Texas and California. Puerto Ricans are concentrated in the New York metropolitan area, and Cubans live primarily in southern Florida. In addition to these general trends, Hispanics are moving to other parts of the United States as well.

The socioeconomic status of Hispanics affects their power in United States society, their self-identity, the quality of their lives, the services available to them, and the opportunities and goods that are achievable. A quite significant gap remains between the socioeconomic status of Hispanics and that of non-Hispanic whites in the United States. In March 1999, Hispanics were engaged in the civilian labor force at about the same rate as non-Hispanic whites (67% and 67.1%, respectively) (Ramírez 2000). However, most Hispanics were in semiskilled and service positions and in fishing, forestry, and farming; most Hispanics were not in managerial or professional positions. The lack of available opportunities, as well as a limited command of English, discrimination, and lower educational status, affects the quality of life of Hispanics in the United States.

As of March 1999, Hispanics were less likely to have a high school diploma than were non-Hispanic whites. Among Hispanics 25 years or older, 27.8% had less than a ninth-grade education, 56.1% had a high school diploma or more, and about 10.9% had graduated from college. In comparison, 4.5% of non-Hispanic whites had less than a ninth-grade education, 87.7% had a high school diploma or more, and 27.7% had graduated from college (Ramírez 2000).

Hispanic people were three times as likely as non-Hispanic whites to be living below the poverty level as of March 1999 (25.6% compared with 8.2%). Children younger than 18 years were about one-half of all Hispanics living in poverty (47.5%), and 23.4% of all people living in poverty in the United States were of Hispanic origin (Ramírez 2000). Hispanics also had an unemployment rate of 6.7%, which was higher than that for non-Hispanic whites (3.6%) (Ramírez 2000).

Some of the data presented so far for Hispanics are summarized in Table 1–2 (Day 1996; Ramírez 2000; U.S. Bureau of the Census 2000). There are differences among groups of Hispanics in the statistics presented, and the reader is referred for further details to Casas and Vasquez (1996) and Ramírez (2000).

CULTURAL CHARACTERISTICS

Hispanics in general share certain cultural values that differ from those of other populations in the United States. Some of these values include

---

Table 1–2.   Demographics of Hispanics in the United States

There are 35.3 million Hispanics, representing 12.5% of the total population.

Hispanics may be the largest minority in the United States by 2010.

The Hispanic population is made up of 65.2% Mexican Americans, 14.3% Central and South Americans, 9.6% Puerto Ricans, 4.3% Cubans, and 6.6% other Hispanics.

Hispanics are engaged in the civilian labor force at the same rate as non-Hispanic whites.

Hispanics are less likely to have a high school diploma than are non-Hispanic whites.

Poverty is three times more common among Hispanics than among non-Hispanic whites.

Source.   Day 1996; Ramírez 2000; U.S. Bureau of the Census 2000.

- *Familismo,* the strong identification with and attachment to the nuclear and extended family, with a sense of loyalty and duty to the family (Triandis et al. 1982)
- Respect for elderly people and for those in positions of power
- A more traditional sense of gender roles as compared with non-Hispanic whites, including *machismo* (the ideal of the strong, powerful, active man) and *marianismo* (the ideal of the submissive, obedient woman) among certain subgroups
- Collectivism, which emphasizes the needs, objectives, and goals of the group as being more important than those of the individual member of the group (Hofstede 1980)
- *Simpatía,* the avoidance of direct anger and confrontation between people so that relationships can flow smoothly and nicely

These cultural values are generalizations and should be evaluated in the context of other variables that apply to the Hispanic individual; these are discussed in further detail in Chapter 3 of this book.

MENTAL HEALTH OF HISPANICS IN THE UNITED STATES

Research on the mental health of Latinos has been sparse, and more effort is needed to further clarify mental health issues in Hispanic populations. One of the most important psychiatric epidemiologic surveys was the Epidemiologic Catchment Area (ECA) study, in which researchers arrived at various psychiatric diagnoses by using DSM-III (American Psychiatric Association 1980) criteria (Regier et al. 1984). Results of the ECA study showed that African Americans reported somewhat higher rates of any disorder, with substantially higher rates of phobias, schizophrenia, and cognitive impairment, than did other groups. Hispanics had very high scores on depression and alcohol abuse or dependence (Holzer et al. 1995). Table 1–3 illustrates some of the differences in psychiatric disorders between whites, blacks, and Hispanics.

The Los Angeles area was the only site for the ECA study where significant numbers of Hispanics were interviewed and assessed, and most of these Hispanics were Mexican American. The results showed that the prevalence of major depression was similar in Mexican Americans and non-Hispanic whites (Burnam et al. 1987). The ECA data also showed a higher lifetime prevalence for DSM-III dysthymia, panic disorder, and phobia among Mexican American women older than 40 years compared with both non-Hispanic white women older than 40 and Mexican American women younger than 40 years (Karno et al. 1987). This higher vulnerability of Mexican American women older than 40 years to phobias and depressive disorders may be related to numerous psychosocial stressors, which include low educational levels, high unemployment rates, social isolation, financial and domestic strain, stresses of immigration, acculturation issues, and low socioeconomic status. The ECA data also reported that Mexican Americans sought outpatient psychiatric care less often than did non-Hispanic whites and that Mexican Americans in whom a mental disorder had recently been diagnosed were half as likely as non-Hispanic whites to have made a mental health visit (Hough et al. 1987).

Table 1–3. Weighted rates of psychiatric disorder by ethnicity per 100

Psychiatric disorder	White (n=11,900)	Hispanic (n=1,428)	Black (n=4,190)
Any disorder	10.4	11.7	11.9
Alcohol	4.5	6.2	4.8
Depression	2.8	3.1	2.9
Schizophrenia	0.9	0.4	1.5
Phobias	7.9	7.7	13.7
Cognitive impairment	0.9	1.4	3.2

Source.   Holzer et al. 1995.

The ECA data also found that the risk of suicide attempts was higher for those Hispanics who had major depression than for those Hispanics who had other psychiatric diagnoses. In the Los Angeles ECA study, the rate of suicidal ideation reported by Hispanics was about half that reported by non-Hispanic whites (8.8% vs. 18.9%), and the rate of suicide attempts reported by Hispanics was approximately two-thirds that reported by non-Hispanic whites (3.2% vs. 5.1%) (Sorenson and Golding 1988a). These data are consistent with other studies that found a suicide rate for Hispanics about one-half of that for non-Hispanic whites (Sorenson and Golding 1988b). The ECA data also found that 1) both Hispanic and non-Hispanic white women reported more suicide attempts than did men of either ethnic group, 2) divorced or separated individuals had higher rates of suicidal ideation and suicide attempts in both ethnic groups, 3) Hispanics of higher educational status were at higher risk for suicidal ideation and suicide attempts than were less educated Hispanics, and 4) the risk of a suicide attempt was increased seven times by the presence of a psychiatric disorder, especially major depression (Sorenson and Golding 1988a). Possible explanations for the lower suicidal ideation and suicide attempts among Hispanics than among non-Hispanic whites include stronger cultural ties among Hispanics, a higher participation of Hispanics in religious and other social activities, Catholicism and its prohibition against suicide, and religious commitment to the Catholic church (Sorenson and Golding 1988b). Some of the findings from the ECA study for Hispanics are summarized in Table 1–4.

Table 1–4.   Epidemiologic Catchment Area study psychiatric findings for Hispanics

High prevalence of major depression was similar to that of non-Hispanic whites.

High rate of alcohol abuse and dependence was found.

Lifetime prevalence of dysthymia, panic disorder, and phobias was higher among Mexican American women older than 40 years than among all other groups.

Hispanics were less likely to seek outpatient psychiatric care and to visit a mental health professional for their problems than were non-Hispanic whites.

Source.   Burnam et al. 1987; Karno et al. 1987.

Another study, the National Comorbidity Study, found that the rate of major depression was much greater for Hispanics than for non-Hispanic whites over a 30-day period (Blazer et al. 1994). This study found that 8.1% of the Hispanics had major depressive episodes compared with 4.7% of the non-

Hispanic whites over a 30-day period. Lifetime percentage of major depressive episodes was similar at about 18% (Blazer et al. 1994). Some of the reasons for the prevalence of major depression in the Hispanic community may be the possible effects of immigration and acculturation, social isolation, low socioeconomic status, and low educational level—all factors that have been associated with persistent depressed mood (Golding and Lipton 1990).

Despite the high prevalence of major depression in the Hispanic community, the problem is still not adequately recognized. Muñoz and colleagues (1990) found that 44% of 100 Hispanic patients randomly questioned at a public health clinic in San Diego, California, had mild to severe major depression and that none of them had received treatment for depression. Furthermore, they found that the physicians at the clinic were not aware, nor did they suspect, that these patients' somatic complaints might have been a manifestation of major depressive disorders (Muñoz et al. 1990).

Some of the possible reasons for the missed diagnosis of major depression in Hispanics may include the tendency for some Hispanics to somatize rather than present with psychological problems, the lack of access to mental health resources, language and cultural barriers between patients and providers, and the stigma of mental illness in the Hispanic community. Some Hispanic patients may express their distress in a somatic way and may complain of upset stomach, headache, and other somatic symptoms. Evidence shows that Latin Americans with major depression present with more somatic symptoms than do their North American counterparts, especially Latin Americans from more traditional backgrounds and lower socioeconomic status (Escobar et al. 1983; Mezzich and Raab 1980). This tendency for greater somatization among Hispanics may have many causes, some of which might include the attempt to legitimize care-seeking behavior and the wish to avoid the stigma associated with mental illness and psychological problems. Frequent idioms of distress, such as *nervios,* may be misunderstood and misdiagnosed by clinicians not familiar with Hispanic culture. The term *nervios* represents a global expression of distress that might be best translated as "upset and nervous." Hispanic patients may present with somatic complaints that may mask a diagnosis of major depression or anxiety disorders, and they need to be evaluated for depressive and other psychiatric disorders in addition to medical conditions. Alcohol and substance abuse as they affect Latinos will be discussed in detail in Chapter 14 of this book.

The results of studies that have tried to determine whether the prevalence of mental health problems differs between Hispanics and non-Hispanics have been inconsistent and inconclusive. Some studies have concluded that Hispanics do have higher rates of disorders than do other ethnic groups (Shrout et al. 1992), whereas others have found the opposite. Several factors add to the confusion about this issue: there has been a paucity of research on the relation between psychiatric epidemiology and ethnicity; each of the studies had a different population, with different numbers and methodology; there may have been biases in reporting; the definition of who is considered Hispanic was unclear; and the studies did not take into account the considerable heterogeneity among Hispanics.

Rogler and colleagues (1989) developed hypotheses that may explain the discrepancy in study results. They noted that studies that showed more psychiatric disorders among Hispanics than among other groups used symptoms to define these disorders, whereas the studies that showed no difference in psychiatric disorders between Hispanics and other groups relied mostly on discrete psychiatric diagnoses (Rogler et al. 1989). Perhaps Hispanics have many psychological complaints and issues but not enough to warrant formal psychiatric diagnoses from a structured interview for psychiatric disorders. Rogler et al. suggested that both a structured interview and a symptom checklist should be used to clarify diagnoses.

There are also questions about the applicability of DSM-III, DSM-IV (American Psychiatric Association 1994), and other diagnostic systems to the study of Hispanics. Even though a cultural formulation is included in DSM-IV and is a part of every mental health assessment, there still may be a bias toward diagnosing populations on the basis of North American (primarily non-Hispanic white) population samples. The DSM-IV diagnostic criteria may not be entirely applicable to Hispanics. Escobar and colleagues (1987) examined the prevalence of somatization disorder symptoms elicited with the Diagnostic Interview Schedule in the Los Angeles ECA study and compared the mean number of somatization symptoms based on gender, age, and ethnicity in Mexican American and non-Hispanic white populations. A less restrictive operational definition of somatization than the DSM-III criteria was used, and 4.4% of the respondents met criteria for the abridged cutoff score of somatization, whereas only 0.03% of the respondents met the full DSM-III criteria for somatization disorder. Hispanic women older than 40 years had a higher mean number of symptoms than did any other group; also, Mexican American women older than 40 who had lower acculturation levels tended to somatize more than did Mexican American women older than 40 who were more acculturated to the United States (Escobar et al. 1987). Therefore, some Hispanic groups have higher rates of somatization symptoms that may not be detected if only the full DSM criteria are applied to epidemiologic studies.

Villaseñor and Waitzkin (1999) examined the limitations of the Composite International Diagnostic Interview (CIDI) in the assessment of somatization among Hispanic patients. Developed by the World Health Organization and the U.S. National Institute of Mental Health, the CIDI grew from and eventually supplanted the Diagnostic Interview Schedule, which was used for the ECA studies. Villaseñor and Waitzkin found that the CIDI led to inaccurate identification of somatoform symptoms in Hispanic patients as the result of language differences between patients and physicians, cultural syndromes of Hispanic patients that were not recognized by Western medicine, and financial obstacles to the access of health care.

Holzer and colleagues (1995) found that the low socioeconomic status of Latinos predisposed them to an increased prevalence of psychiatric disorders compared with non-Hispanic whites but that low socioeconomic status was not the only reason for this increased prevalence in Latinos.

Few psychiatric epidemiologic studies of Hispanics have been done, and even fewer have compared Hispanics from different countries or origins in terms of prevalence rates for psychiatric disorders. Shrout and colleagues (1992) conducted a statistical analysis of comparable survey designs of psychiatric disorder prevalence. One study was of Puerto Ricans and the other of Mexican Americans (immigrants and United States natives) and non-Hispanic whites in the Los Angeles area. Mexican American immigrants had lower rates of psychiatric disorders than did the other groups, and Mexican American natives and non-Hispanic whites had higher rates of alcohol abuse and affective symptoms than did the Puerto Ricans.

Several explanations could account for the differing prevalence of mental disorders among Mexican American immigrants, Mexican American natives, and Puerto Ricans in Puerto Rico. Acculturation may have played a role in this difference. Another explanation is that those Mexican Americans who were in the immigrant group had to overcome the obstacles of immigration to the United States and the stresses associated with it; therefore, they may have represented a self-selected sample of people who survived the rigorous process of immigration to the United States. The Mexican American immigrants may have been thankful for being able to be in the United States, whereas those Mexican Americans born in the United States perhaps had no frame of reference for how difficult life was or must have been in Mexico, which may have led to more affective disorders and alcoholism among them. This may also explain why Mexican American natives would have higher rates of psychiatric disorders than Puerto Ricans, because the Mexican American natives were a minority population that experienced a lot of stress, whereas Puerto Ricans represented the majority population on their island and spoke their native language.

HISTORY OF HISPANICS IN THE UNITED STATES

Hispanics in the United States come from various backgrounds and circumstances. Most Latinos are descendants of several groups: Spaniards who came to the Americas, indigenous populations before the Spaniards' arrival, and black people from Africa. This mixture has given rise to the different groups in the Hispanic population: *mestizo* (Spanish and American Indian), *mulato* (Spanish and black), and *zambo* (American Indian and black).

By the early sixteenth century, Spanish explorers were already colonizing various regions of the United States, especially Florida and the Southwest. In the early nineteenth century, Spain sold Florida to the United States and gave Louisiana to the French. Most countries in Central and South America achieved independence from Spain in the 1810s and 1820s.

After the 1846–1848 Mexican War and the 1848 Treaty of Guadalupe-Hidalgo, Mexico ceded almost half of its territory to the United States, which included the present-day states of Texas, Colorado, California, Arizona, and New Mexico. The Mexicans who were living in Mexico at that time found themselves now living within a new country with new rules and with the added weight of discrimination; they were colonized by the non-Hispanic whites. Many of the original inhabitants of the United States Southwest were Mexicans who lost lands and whatever privileges they may have had as Mexicans and were incorporated into the United States through colonization and subjugation. Many of their descendants who still live in the Southwest continue to experience a sense of betrayal and loss of their original land.

Non-Hispanic whites employed Mexicans within the agriculture, mining, and railroad industries after the expansion of capital toward the West and increasing settlements. More job opportunities arose in the 1880s with an increasing wave of migration from Mexico to the United States between 1880 and 1929. Another factor that contributed to increased migration during that time was the Mexican Revolution (1910–1917) and the migration north to try to find better opportunities. After the economic depression beginning in 1929, the United States restricted the entry of Mexicans into the country, but this situation changed during World War II, when the United States needed additional agricultural labor and instituted the *bracero* program, which allowed Mexicans to work in the United States. Most of the workers in the agriculture, industry, and service fields were hired as cheap labor and experienced social and economic disadvantages, with low salaries, poor job protection, and poor job stability. Since World War II, the Mexican American population experienced advances in education, income, and political efficacy. Most of them continue to live in the cities within the Southwest but with a greater degree of assimilation into non-Hispanic white society. Many have moved away from Spanish as a primary language, and the isolation of the barrio has declined. A disproportionate overrepresentation of Mexicans and Mexican Americans within the field of agriculture as seasonal and permanent laborers remains.

After Spain lost the Spanish-American War (1898), Puerto Rico became a United States territory; it later became a commonwealth (1952). Most Puerto Ricans only started migrating in increasing numbers to the United States in the 1950s as a result of rapid industrialization within the island and increasing unemployment. The absence of immigration restrictions, the cheap air travel between Puerto Rico and the United States, and the increasing numbers of family members in the United States also promoted this migration; most Puerto Ricans went to New York City. They worked in unskilled, blue-collar jobs, primarily in the manufacturing and service industries. The 1960s and 1970s saw a return migration to Puerto Rico that decreased during the 1980s. Because so many Puerto Ricans have familial ties in both New York and Puerto Rico, they tend to fly back and forth between the two countries.

The Puerto Rican identity is shaped by the island's relationship to the United States. Some Puerto Ricans want to achieve independence from the United States and become an independent nation, whereas others want to remain a commonwealth, and still others would like to effect a compromise. Many Puerto Ricans have a sense of not being one or the other, not really being from the United States but also not belonging to an independent state.

Cubans started immigrating to the United States, especially to Miami, Florida, in large numbers after the 1959 revolution and the takeover of Cuba by Fidel Castro. The first wave of immigrants was made up of the elite upper classes who could leave with their wealth and possessions and reestablish themselves in Miami. Middle-class professionals and blue-collar workers, some of whom had all their possessions confiscated, followed them. Several waves of migration of Cubans to Dade County, Florida, occurred until the early 1970s, when the Cuban government imposed restrictions on migration to the United States. Later waves of migration tended to be made up of younger and less-educated people. Another large migration of the *marielitos* (named after the port of Mariel in Cuba, from which they left) occurred in 1980.

Most Cubans live in Miami; some live in New Jersey and New York and in each of the states in the United States. The Cubans usually present with a higher socioeconomic status than the Puerto Ricans and Mexican Americans, for several reasons: their immigration was political, not economic; more professionals and upper- and middle-class people migrated to the United States within the Cuban group; the Cubans did not come here to be hired as cheap labor (as the Puerto Ricans and Mexican Americans did); and in many cases Cubans received assistance from the United States government and other forms of help to achieve the kinds of jobs they were performing in Cuba. Moreover, most early immigrants were granted legal immigration status.

Several other groups of Latinos have come to the United States from other countries during the past two decades. Civil wars, revolutions, and political upheaval in many Central American countries during the past 15 years (El Salvador, Nicaragua, Guatemala, the Dominican Republic) and the recent devastation after Hurricane Mitch in 1998 have led to large numbers of inhabitants of these countries continuing to immigrate or attempting to immigrate to the United States. The immigration trends for these other groups are discussed further in the chapters of this book discussing individual countries and their people (Part II).

CONCLUSIONS

We have presented a brief overview of the Latino population in the United States. Because Hispanics are expected to soon be the largest minority group in the country, it is imperative that mental health practitioners become familiar with the basic characteristics of the Hispanic peoples. It is hoped that the new century will bring increasing knowledge about this critical and evolving population.

REFERENCES

American Psychiatric Association: Diagnostic and Statistical Manual of Mental Disorders, 3rd Edition. Washington, DC, American Psychiatric Association, 1980

American Psychiatric Association: Diagnostic and Statistical Manual of Mental Disorders, 4th Edition. Washington, DC, American Psychiatric Association, 1994

Blazer DG, Kessler RC, McGonagle KA, et al: The prevalence and distribution of major depression in a national community sample: the National Comorbidity Survey. Am J Psychiatry 151:979–986, 1994

Burnam MA, Hough RL, Escobar JI, et al: Six-month prevalence of specific psychiatric disorders among Mexican Americans and non-Hispanic whites in Los Angeles. Arch Gen Psychiatry 44:687–694, 1987

Casas MT, Vasquez M: Counseling the Hispanic, in Counseling Across Cultures, 4th Edition. Edited by Pedersen P, Lonner WJ, Draguns J, et al. Thousand Oaks, CA, Sage, 1996, pp 146–176

Day JC: Population Projections of the United States by Age, Sex, Race, and Hispanic Origin: 1995 to 2050. U.S. Bureau of the Census, Current Population Reports, P25-1130. Washington, DC, U.S. Government Printing Office, 1996

Escobar JI, Gomez J, Tuason VB: Depressive phenomenology in North and South American patients. Am J Psychiatry 140:47–51, 1983

Escobar JI, Burnam MA, Karno M, et al: Somatization in the community. Arch Gen Psychiatry 44:713–718, 1987

Golding JM, Lipton RI: Depressed mood and major depressive disorder in two ethnic groups. J Psychiatr Res 24:65–82, 1990

Hayes-Bautista D, Chapa J: Latino terminology: conceptual bases for standardized terminology. Am J Public Health 73:274–276, 1987

Hofstede G: Culture's Consequences. Beverly Hills, CA, Sage, 1980

Holzer CE, Swanson J-W, Shea BM: Ethnicity, social status, and psychiatric disorder in the Epidemiologic Catchment Area Survey, in Social Psychiatry Across Cultures: Studies From North America, Asia, Europe, and Africa. Edited by Price RK, Shea BM, Mookherjee HN. New York, Plenum, 1995, pp 93–104

Hough RL, Landsverk JA, Karno M, et al: Utilization of health and mental health services by Los Angeles Mexican Americans and non-Hispanic whites. Arch Gen Psychiatry 44:695–701, 1987

Karno M, Hough RL, Burnam MA, et al: Lifetime prevalence of specific psychiatric disorders among Mexican Americans and non-Hispanic whites in Los Angeles. Arch Gen Psychiatry 44:695–701, 1987

Mezzich JE, Raab ES: Depressive symptomatology across the Americas. Arch Gen Psychiatry 37:818–823, 1980

Muñoz RA, Boddy P, Prime R, et al: Depression in the Hispanic community. Ann Clin Psychiatry 2:115–120, 1990

Pérez-Stable E: Issues in Latino health care. West J Med 146:213–218, 1987

Ramírez RR: The Hispanic Population in the United States: March 1999. U.S. Bureau of the Census, P20-527. Washington, DC, U.S. Government Printing Office, 2000

Regier DA, Myers JK, Kramer M, et al: The NIMH Catchment Area Program. Arch Gen Psychiatry 41:934–948, 1984

Rogler LH, Malgady RG, Rodriguez O: Hispanics and Mental Health: A Framework for Research. Malabar, FL, RE Krieger, 1989

Shrout PE, Canino GJ, Bird HR, et al: Mental health status among Puerto Ricans, Mexican Americans, and non-Hispanic whites. Am J Community Psychol 20:729–752, 1992

Sorenson SB, Golding JM: Suicide ideation and attempts in Hispanics and non-Hispanic whites: demographic and psychiatric disorder issues. Suicide Life Threat Behav 18:205–218, 1988a

Sorenson SB, Golding JM: Prevalence of suicide attempts in a Mexican-American population: prevention implications of immigration and cultural issues. Suicide Life Threat Behav 18:322–333, 1988b

Triandis HC, Marín G, Betancourt H, et al: Dimensions of Familism Among Hispanic and Mainstream Navy Recruits. Chicago, University of Illinois, 1982

U.S. Bureau of the Census: 1990 Census of Population: Persons of Hispanic Origin in the United States. Washington, DC, U.S. Government Printing Office, 1993

U.S. Bureau of the Census: Census 2000 Redistricting Data (PL 94-171). Summary File for states, Tables PL1, PL2, PL3, and PL4. Washington, DC, U.S. Government Printing Office, 2001

Valdivieso R, Davis C: U.S. Hispanics: Challenging Issues for the 1990s. Washington, DC, Population Reference Bureau, 1988

Villaseñor Y, Waitzkin H: Limitations of a structured psychiatric diagnostic instrument in assessing somatization among Latino patients in primary care. Med Care 37:637–646, 1999

CHAPTER 2

Physical Health Status of Latinos in the United States

Eliseo J. Pérez-Stable, M.D.

Anna M. Nápoles-Springer, Ph.D.

THE HEALTH STATUS OF Latinos often has been referred to as an epidemiologic paradox. On the basis of the lower socioeconomic status of Latinos compared with non-Latino whites (henceforth called whites), one would predict higher indicators of morbidity and mortality for most diseases. Despite major barriers to health care, including lack of access to primary care and less preventive care, epidemiologic data indicate that Latinos have a better health profile for the leading causes of death (heart disease, cancer, and cerebrovascular diseases) than do whites. National surveys indicate that this finding may be attributable to lifestyle factors, which may be culturally influenced, such as lower smoking rates. Nonetheless, Latinos continue to be disproportionately affected by selected conditions such as human immunodeficiency virus (HIV) infection, diabetes mellitus, cirrhosis of the liver, homicides, and cancers of the cervix, liver, gallbladder, and stomach. Much of this disproportionate burden of disease is associated with the lack of access to preventive health care and early treatment services. However, precise information on morbidity and mortality rates for Latinos as an ethnic group has been systematically collected

This work was supported by Public Health Service grant HSO7373-01 from the Agency for Health Care Policy and Research.

only in the past two decades, and underestimation of population denominators also may distort reported rates. In this chapter, we present an overview of available national data on indicators of mortality and morbidity, with an emphasis on conditions that disproportionately affect Latinos. We then discuss awareness of prevention issues and risk behaviors, with a special emphasis on nicotine addiction, attitudes toward physicians and medical care, seeking help for medical care, and barriers to medical care.

MORTALITY

Age-adjusted death rates in Latino men and women are about 25% lower than those in their white counterparts. The overall age-adjusted death rates for Latino men and women in 1998 were 442.7 and 255.5 per 100,000, respectively, compared with 595.9 and 379.0 per 100,000 for non-Latino men and women, respectively. Death rates for Latinos ranged from 203.1 per 100,000 for Cuban women to 540.8 for Puerto Rican men (Murphy 2000).

Seven of the 10 leading causes of death were the same for Latinos and non-Latino whites (heart disease, cancer, accidents, cerebrovascular disease, diabetes mellitus, pneumonia and influenza, and chronic obstructive pulmonary disease) (Murphy 2000). Homicides, chronic liver disease, and perinatal conditions were included in the 10 leading causes of death for Latinos but not for the total non-Latino population. In 1998, age-adjusted death rates due to heart disease, cerebrovascular disease, and malignant neoplasms were more than three times higher for non-Latinos than for Latinos (Murphy 2000). Diabetes was the fourth leading cause of death among Latina women and sixth among Latino men, whereas it ranked seventh for non-Latino men and women (Murphy 2000). The mortality rate from diabetes in women aged 45 to 64 was more than three times higher for Latina women than for non-Latina women (65.6 vs. 19.6 per 100,000) (Murphy 2000).

Deaths due to homicide and HIV infection ranked higher for Latinos than for non-Latinos between ages 25 and 44 years (Murphy 2000). HIV infection and chronic liver disease also ranked higher for the Latino population than for the total non-Latino population for ages 45–64 years (Murphy 2000).

MORBIDITY

Diabetes Mellitus

According to the 1988–1994 National Health and Nutrition Examination Survey III (NHANES III), the prevalence of diabetes is 1.8 times higher in Mexican Americans than in whites (20.3% vs. 11.2%) (Harris et al. 1998a).

The influence of indigenous and African admixture has been hypothesized as accounting for the disproportionate rate of diabetes among Latinos. Rates of diabetes in Mexican Americans have increased 17% since the 1982–1984 Hispanic Health and Nutrition Examination Survey (HHANES) (Harris et al. 1998a). These findings are consistent with data from the Behavioral Risk Factor Surveillance System (BRFSS) for 1990–1998, which reflect a 38% increase in the prevalence of diabetes among Latinos (Mokdad et al. 2000). The age- and sex-standardized prevalence of undiagnosed diabetes also was higher in Mexican Americans than in whites (4.2% vs. 2.5%) (Harris et al. 1998a).

A major problem that contributes to excess morbidity and secondary complications due to diabetes in Latinos is their greater likelihood of receiving a diagnosis and treatment when the disease is more advanced. In fact, compared with whites, Latinos with diabetes were less likely to report preventive care to detect diabetes-related complications. For example, Latinos were less likely to have documented dilated eye examinations (59.6% vs. 54.1%), foot examinations (56.2% vs. 46.8%), self-monitoring of blood glucose (48.1% vs. 34.8%), and glycosylated hemoglobin tests (26.5% vs. 17.6%) (Centers for Disease Control and Prevention 2000a). Prevalence of diabetic retinopathy was 84% higher in Mexican Americans than in whites in those previously diagnosed with diabetes (Harris et al. 1998b). A study of hospitalizations for lower-extremity amputations in south Texas found that diabetes caused a higher proportion of amputations among Mexican Americans than among whites (85.9% vs. 56.3%) (Lavery et al. 1999). Additionally, Mexican Americans are at higher risk for developing proteinuria and end-stage renal disease (Pugh 1996). The severity of these problems points to the importance of encouraging health care access and care seeking among Latinos, as well as preventive measures that may reduce their risk of developing diabetes, such as engaging in physical activity, maintaining ideal body weight, and developing healthy nutritional habits. The HHANES study showed that 24% of the Mexican Americans, 40% of the Puerto Ricans, and 58% of the Cubans who had diabetes were unaware that they had the disease (Flegal et al. 1991).

Hypertension

Age-adjusted rates of hypertension declined substantially in whites aged 20–74 years between 1976–1980 and 1988–1994 (from 43.9% to 24.4% in men and from 32.1% to 19.3% in women) (National Center for Health Statistics 2000). These rates reflect the total prevalence during each of the 4- to 6-year data collection cycles. However, hypertension rates among Mexican Americans remained essentially the same during the same periods, with a total age-adjusted prevalence rate of 25.2% for men and 22.0% for women in a 1988–1994 survey (National Center for Health Statistics 2000). Latinos are less likely than whites to have their blood pressure under control (Pavlik et al. 1996). Progress toward awareness, treatment, and control of hypertension in Latinos requires increasing attention to community awareness, facilitating access to care for this group, and sensitizing clinicians.

Cancer

Cancer incidence and mortality rates are generally lower for Latinos than for whites. The age-adjusted death rate for malignant neoplasms in 1996–1998 was 92.3 and 65.3 per 100,000 for Latino men and women, respectively, compared with 148.8 and 105.9 per 100,000 for white men and women, respectively (National Center for Health Statistics 2000). The leading causes of cancer death for both Latinos and whites—which include lung, breast, colon, and prostate cancers—are substantially less common among Latinos (Ries et al. 2000). For most types of cancers, the incidence rate for Latinos is lower than that for whites. However, relative to white men, Latino men have higher rates of stomach cancer (1.6 times greater) and liver cancer (2.2 times greater). Relative to white women, Latina women have higher rates of cancer of the cervix (2.2 times greater), liver (2.0 times greater), stomach (2.1 times greater), and gallbladder (3.3 times greater) (Canto and Chu 2000). The lower rates most likely result from dietary habits, less smoking, and cultural and biological factors that have yet to be elucidated. Despite these lower rates, lung, breast, colon, and prostate cancer continue to be the most common among Latinos, and for both breast and colon cancers, recommended early detection tests need to be promoted in this group. Limited data from regional registries show that 5-year survival rates for colorectal, lung, breast, and prostate cancer are actually lower for Mexican Americans than for whites, which could be related to diagnosis at later stages of disease and disparities in access to or quality of treatment services (Zambrana et al. 1999).

AIDS

Although the proportion of AIDS cases among whites has decreased over time, the proportion among Latinos has increased (Division of HIV/AIDS Prevention 2000). In 1991, surveillance data indicated that 52% of AIDS cases in U.S. adults were in whites and 17% were in Latinos (Centers for Disease Control 1991). In 1999, by comparison, 32% of AIDS cases were in whites and 19% were in Latinos (Division of HIV/AIDS Prevention 2000). In Latino men, having sex with men (39.0% of reported cases) and injection drug use (33.5% of reported cases) are both important risk factors for HIV infection. In Latina women, the primary risk factors are injection drug use (42.5% of reported cases) and heterosexual contact (38.9%) (National Center for Health Statistics 2000). The rate of pediatric (younger than 13 years) AIDS cases in 1999 was somewhat higher in Latinos than in whites (0.8 vs. 0.1 per 100,000) (National Center for Health Statistics 2000).

PREVENTIVE HEALTH BEHAVIORS AND RISK FACTORS

Nicotine Addiction

Cigarette smoking is the leading cause of preventable morbidity and mortality in the United States among all ethnic groups. National and regional surveys have found that on average Latinos smoke at lower rates than do whites and that among current smokers, Latinos smoke fewer cigarettes per day than do these other groups. Data from the 1997 National Health Interview Survey (NHIS) showed that the overall prevalence of current cigarette smoking was lower for Latinos (20.4%) than for whites (25.3%), although rates vary substantially by sex (Centers for Disease Control and Prevention 1999). For Latino men, the rates are approaching those of white men (26.2% vs. 27.4%), whereas for Latina women, the rates are low relative to white women (14.3% vs. 23.3%) (Centers for Disease Control and Prevention 1999). In the United States, from 1988 to 1995, the number of Latinos who reported being current smokers increased from 2.8 to 3.2 million. Concurrently, the number of Latinos who reported quitting decreased from 2.2 to 2.0 million, and the number of Latinos who have never smoked increased from 6.8 to 11.5 million (Centers for Disease Control and Prevention 2000c). For those who reported smoking every day, more than 20% of the whites reported smoking 21 or more cigarettes per day compared with 7% of the Latinos. For those who reported that they do not smoke every day, 83.4% of the Latinos reported smoking 5 or fewer cigarettes per day compared with 65.5% of the whites (Division of Adult and Community Health 1995–1999). During the 1990s, smoking rates increased among high school students in general (Centers for Disease Control and Prevention 2000). Data from a national survey conducted in 1999 indicated that 11.0% of middle-school Latino students (vs. 8.8% of white students) and 25.8% of high-school Latino students (vs. 32.8% of white students) smoked cigarettes (Centers for Disease Control and Prevention 2000c).

The level of acculturation as measured by a short language-based scale (Marín et al. 1987) appears to influence smoking behavior among Mexican

American and Central American Latinos (Marín et al. 1989; Pérez-Stable et al. 1998). Smoking rates were higher for the more acculturated Latino women but lower for the more acculturated men (Marín et al. 1989). These data suggest that smoking behavior among Latinos becomes more similar to that of whites with increasing levels of acculturation and, as a consequence, that smoking may become a more serious problem for Latino women. When one considers current smoking trends among Latino youth and the adverse effects of acculturation on smoking, increased tobacco-related disease morbidity among Latinos will be a concern in the future (U.S. Department of Health and Human Services 1998).

Latino smokers, especially Mexican Americans, reported smoking an average of 8 and 12 cigarettes per day for women and men, respectively (U.S. Department of Health and Human Services 1998). This number is substantially less than the average 19.1 and 23.4 cigarettes per day reported by white women and men, respectively (U.S. Department of Health and Human Services 1998). Although a lower proportion of highly acculturated Latino men smoke, they reported a greater number of cigarettes per day than less acculturated men (Marín et al. 1989). Among women, a higher proportion smoked, and they reported smoking more cigarettes per day as acculturation level increased (Marín et al. 1989). To some extent, Latinos underreport the consumption of cigarettes per day, but even after adjusting for a 20%–25% rate of underreporting among light smokers, Latinos are lighter smokers than whites; this finding is supported by biochemical studies (Pérez-Stable et al. 1990a, 1992a, 1995; Wells et al. 1998). These observations have important implications for cessation strategies because compared with heavy smokers, light smokers are more likely to successfully quit smoking with appropriate motivational messages and self-help methods (U.S. Department of Health and Human Services 1998).

A strong epidemiologic and clinical association is found between smoking and significant depressive symptoms and clinical depression. It is believed that some people may treat their depressed moods with nicotine. An association between cigarette smoking and significant depressive symptoms has been found in Latinos; an odds ratio (OR) of 1.7 (95% confidence interval [CI] = 1.3–2.2) for significant depressive symptoms was reported for current smokers compared with former smokers (OR = 1.1; 95% CI = 0.8–1.6) and never smokers (reference group) (Pérez-Stable et al. 1990b). The interaction of nicotine dependence with significant depressive symptoms, and how this interaction affects cessation, needs further study at both the individual and the community level (Marín and Pérez-Stable 1995).

Most cigarette smokers who successfully quit do so on their own, motivated by a variety of psychological, social, and health-related reasons. Policies regulating smoking, media campaigns against smoking, well-designed self-help cessation materials, and advice from clinicians are potential elements of a public health strategy to promote nonsmoking. Given the substantial differences that exist in sociocultural backgrounds among ethnic groups in the United States, it is reasonable to postulate that ethnic differences in cigarette smoking behavior, attitudes, and beliefs should influence the content of smoking cessation intervention strategies. Studies have shown that, compared with whites, Latinos are less likely to smoke due to habitual cues; as likely to smoke due to emotional cues; and more likely to want to quit because of cigarette smoke's effects on others' health, interpersonal relationships, and their own health (Marín et al. 1990; Pérez-Stable et al. 1998). Latinos are also more likely than whites to report quitting smoking for at least 1 day in the previous year (63% vs. 51%) (Pérez-Stable et al. 1998). These data imply that culturally appropriate public health interventions may be an effective method of promoting smoking cessation among Latino smokers.

Obesity and Physical Activity

Excess body weight appears to place Mexican Americans at higher risk than whites for certain diseases such as diabetes and cardiovascular disease. National data indicate that the proportion of the population that is considered overweight (defined as a body mass index≥25) has grown for both Latinos and whites over the last 20 years (National Center for Health Statistics 2000). Among Mexican Americans aged 20–74 years, combined age-adjusted data for 1988–1994 showed that 67.0% of the men and 67.8% of the women were considered overweight (vs. 59.9% of white men and 45.7% of white women) (National Center for Health Statistics 2000). The same trend has been observed in children and adolescents aged 6–17 years. Approximately 15.8% and 14.8% of Mexican American girls and boys, respectively, were found to be overweight based on combined data for 1988–1994 (compared with 11.9% and 11.8% of white girls and boys, respectively) (National Center for Health Statistics 2000). An analysis of NHANES III data found that after adjusting for age, education, percentage of energy from dietary fat, leisure-time physical activity, and smoking, waist circumference was significantly greater in United States–born Mexican men and women than in Mexican-born men and women. This study also found that United States–born Mexican women who spoke English had a significantly greater waist circumference than United States–born Mexican women who spoke Spanish (Sundquist and Winkleby 2000). These results point to the effects of birthplace and acculturation on the development of obesity. Latinos in general appear to report lower levels of leisure-time physical activity than do whites, with 33.9% of Latinos and 22.3% of whites reporting sedentary lifestyles. However, a larger proportion of Latinos also reported 5 hours or more of hard occupational activity compared with whites (33.0 vs. 21.9%) (Centers for Disease Control and Prevention 2000b).

Nutrition

According to BRFSS data for 1998, only 22.4% of Latinos reported consuming five or more servings of fruits and vegetables per day on average compared with 24.3% of whites (Division of Adult and Community Health, National Center for Chronic Disease Prevention and Health Promotion et al. 2000). Regional data from Texas and California also showed that Latinos are more likely than are whites to consume saturated fats in the form of whole milk, fried foods, and use of animal fat for cooking and to consume more beans as a highly valued source of fiber (Haffner et al. 1985; Otero-Sabogal et al. 1995).

Hyperlipidemia

The prevalence of high serum cholesterol levels ($\geq$240 mg/dL), based on combined data for 1988–1994 NHANES III, appeared to be similar for white and Mexican American men (17.8% for both groups) and higher for white women than for Latina women (20.2% vs. 17.5%) (National Center for Health Statistics 2000). Compared with whites, Latinos also were less likely to report having ever been told by a doctor that their blood cholesterol is high (24.5% vs. 30.4%) (Division of Adult and Community Health, National Center for Chronic Disease Prevention and Health Promotion et al. 2000). The NHANES III study showed that Mexican Americans are more likely than whites to have a lipid pattern associated with diabetes, hyperinsulinemia, and increased cardiovascular risk (Winkleby et al. 1998). High-density lipoprotein cholesterol is protective against heart disease, and levels are decreased among Mexican Americans with diabetes and elevated triglyceride levels. Total cholesterol levels may be less useful than evaluating the subfractions to accurately determine cardiovascular risk.

Prevention and Health Screening

The relatively young median age of Latinos represents a tremendous opportunity for interventions to increase preventive health practices and to reduce behaviors that increase risk of disease and premature death. Such interventions could result in reductions in chronic illness and morbidity and could eventually lead to decreased mortality. Preventive interventions must be tailored to meet the specific needs of Latino subgroups and to make full use of the community's resources, including the skills and commitment of its people. Improvement of modifiable risk factors such as nutritional habits, alcohol consumption, cigarette smoking, sedentary lifestyle, obtaining health care screenings, and environmental exposures need to be addressed by linguistically, culturally, and educationally appropriate methods. Largely preventable diseases such as invasive cervical cancer, cirrhosis, and lung cancer can be greatly reduced through reductions in associated risk behaviors. In 1998, 11% of Latinos reported an interval of greater than 3 years since their last health care contact compared with 5.0% of whites (National Center for Health Statistics 2000). Among children younger than 18 years, 19.5% of Latinos reported no health care visits within the past 12 months compared with 10.7% of white children (National Center for Health Statistics 2000). Thus, increased access to preventive care and raising awareness of risk reduction strategies among Latinos continue to be important public health concerns.

An analysis of pooled NHIS data on Latina women for 1990 and 1992 provided estimates of cancer screening rates for Latino subgroups (Zambrana et al. 1999). According to this study, the proportion of women aged 18 and older who reported having had a Pap smear in the past 3 years ranged from 72% in Mexican women to 80% in Mexican American women. Seventy-three percent of Cuban women and 77% of Puerto Rican women reported having had a Pap smear in the past 3 years, although these rates were still well below the Healthy People 2000 target of greater than 95% (Zambrana et al. 1999). The proportion of women aged 35 and older who reported having had mammography in the past 3 years ranged from 35% in Mexican women to 54% in Mexican American women. The rates for Cuban and Puerto Rican women were 77% and 83%, respectively (Zambrana et al. 1999). The true prevalence of breast and cervical cancer screening may be lower because these estimates were based on telephone survey methods and excluded poorer households without telephones. These estimates also included women in the denominator for whom recommendation of a specific screening examination (mammography for women younger than 50 years) remains controversial.

SOCIOCULTURAL FACTORS IN THE TREATMENT OF LATINO PATIENTS

Cultural Models of Health and Illness

The provision of culturally competent health care services is assuming primary importance in a nation that is becoming increasingly diverse. The medical encounter occurs in a context that reflects the sociocultural, economic, educational, linguistic, and personal backgrounds of both the physician and the patient. The effectiveness of communication is largely dependent on the physician's ability to bridge differences in background and experience. Vital to the discussion of culturally suitable approaches to the provision of health care services in the Latino population is the acknowledgment of the heterogeneity of that population. Latinos differ in national origin, religion, urbanization, acculturation, language, and education, among other factors. Stereotyping or generalizations can be misleading, and individual differences must be considered in the context of the medical encounter. Thus, medical practitioners treating Latino patients need to be adept at assessing potential areas of congruence and differences in attitudes, beliefs, and expectations that may impede or promote the quality of health care and medical outcomes. During medical encounters, Latinos may make attributions about illness and health that do not fit a biomedical model, which may result in miscommunication, disparities in role expectations, less than optimal care, and inadequate adherence to physician recommendations.

Clinicians need to understand the explanatory models of illnesses that an individual patient uses to conceptualize an illness episode. Latino patients may subscribe to cultural beliefs and practices that influence perceptions of disease etiology, the development of symptoms, reasons for becoming ill, and appropriate methods of diagnosis and treatment. When these beliefs pose a serious threat to the patient's health, these ethnomedical practices should be discouraged in a sensitive and respectful manner. In most cases, these health beliefs are not harmful and can be successfully combined with biomedical interventions and ultimately improve adherence (Pachter 1994). Thus, emphasis should be placed on integrating the physician's explanatory models of illness with those of the Latino patient. A nonjudgmental exploration of the patient's cultural beliefs about the causes and symptoms of illness and any form of self-care should be conducted in a culturally sensitive manner (Pachter 1994). Illnesses such as *empacho, susto,* and *ataque de nervios*[1] should be acknowledged and reviewed with the patient to see how they can be integrated with a biomedical approach.

Cross-cultural differences in presentation of symptoms have been linked to differential rates of somatization, to posttraumatic stress disorder in immigrants and refugees, and to clinical depression (Castillo et al. 1995). Latinos may be at risk for misdiagnosis or inappropriate interventions because of a lack of sensitivity by medical professionals to culturally based somatoform symptoms. Furthermore, Latinos tend to associate a stigma with certain illnesses such as cancer (Pérez-Stable et al. 1992b). Recommendations regarding dietary and other types of behavioral changes must be considered in the light of cultural values and preferences. Care must be taken to recommend dietary changes that are affordable and culturally appropriate.

Interpersonal Communication Preferences

The health care provider should be aware of certain cultural scripts that are commonly held by Latinos. The concept of *simpatía* involves a preference for positive interpersonal relationships characterized by politeness and avoidance of conflict (Triandis et al. 1984). As a result, the physician should be aware that it is not uncommon for a Latino patient to nod assent or indicate agreement when, in fact, he or she has a limited understanding of the issue or may even disagree. This tendency places the burden on the physician to ascertain whether the patient has understood, especially in matters such as taking medications. The clinician should ask the patient to repeat the instructions and reassure the patient that it is perfectly appropriate to ask questions or voice any concerns.

Many Latino patients adhere to the cultural script referred to as *personalismo* (formal friendliness). In busy clinical practices, physicians may operate under time constraints conducive to a directed, businesslike approach to the delivery of health care. For Latinos, the issue of *confianza*, or trust in the medical practitioner, is paramount. Because *personalismo* is a preferred mode for social interactions, Latino patients, in general, may tend to discuss nonmedical issues and routinely inquire about the well-being of the physician and his or her family. A certain amount of self-disclosure on the part of the physician can facilitate an openness and sense of trust on the part of the Latino patient.

Role Expectations

Other beliefs that are commonly adhered to by Latinos include a respect for authority, which is extended to the health care provider. Knowledge, age, ed-

---

[1] *Empacho:* a gastrointestinal syndrome that can include "anorexia, stomachache, vomiting, pain with diarrhea, and generalized abdominal fullness" (Neff 1996, Empacho link). *Susto:* "illness attributed to a frightening event that causes the soul to leave the body and results in unhappiness and sickness.... [and] significant strains in key social roles...it is believed that in extreme cases, susto may result in death" (American Psychiatric Association 2000, p. 903). *Ataque de nervios:* "Commonly reported symptoms include uncontrollable shouting, attacks of crying, trembling, heat in the chest rising into the head, and verbal or physical aggression. [Sometimes includes] dissociative experiences, seizurelike or fainting episodes, and suicidal gestures.... A general feature...is a sense of being out of control" (American Psychiatric Association 2000, p. 899).

ucation, and male gender are considered sources of inherent power, which places people with these characteristics in a hierarchically superior position. Consequently, Latinos often defer to the clinician to make treatment decisions because they view these decisions as the role of the professional. Therefore, the participatory model of medical decision making may be inappropriate for more traditional Latinos. Furthermore, questioning the physician's treatment strategy may be viewed as a lack of respect for the physician, a behavior typically unacceptable to the Latino patient. Clinicians' perceptions of patients from diverse ethnic backgrounds also potentially influence role expectations. In interviews and focus groups conducted with Latino patients, perceived discrimination by health care personnel is frequently cited as a problem.

Gender-based roles are strongly emphasized in traditional Latino culture. A Latino woman is considered largely in her role as mother and caregiver. These beliefs will exert their influence on reproductive health practices. Abortion often is not an option for Latino women, and the use of contraceptive methods may be unacceptable because of religious beliefs, especially in those less acculturated. Female sterilization may be considered a way to facilitate promiscuity by traditional Latino men and thus may lead to objections in treating family members. Latino men are expected to be good family providers, tend to be less communicative than Latina women, and generally are not to display emotion based on a cultural script usually referred to as *machismo*. Sexual behavior is viewed in largely moralistic terms, and double standards are commonly held regarding appropriate sexual behavior. In many Latin American countries, it is acceptable for men to have several sexual partners, including commercial sex workers, whereas women are expected to remain monogamous. In many traditional Latino homes, sexual matters are not openly discussed, and sexual education usually occurs through nonfamilial sources. Often these customs result in inaccurate or incomplete information about sexual anatomy, sexually transmitted diseases, sexual risk factors, and contraception, all contributing to the elevated risk of sexually transmitted diseases, cervical cancer, and teenage pregnancies in Latinos.

Issues of informed consent and advising a patient of a terminal illness are heavily influenced by cultural values and remain controversial. Cultures vary according to their views on death and dying. For Latinos, medical treatment decision making and the delivery of "bad news" often occur in a familial setting. It is also not uncommon for younger family members to protect a terminally ill older spouse or parent by not revealing a terminal illness diagnosis. In fact, a study found that among elderly persons, Mexican Americans employ a family-centered approach to medical decision making when dealing with terminal illness, in contrast to the patient autonomy model preferred by European Americans and African Americans (Blackhall et al. 1995). This study also found that Mexican Americans were less likely to state that the physician should disclose the truth about the diagnosis and prognosis of a terminal illness to the patient than were European Americans and African Americans.

Language Factors

In addition to cultural differences that present unique challenges to non-Latino health care providers, language differences can result in obstacles to the delivery of quality health care. According to the U.S. Bureau of the Census, almost 78% of Latinos speak Spanish at home, and only half report an ability to speak English very well. Language differences present major barriers to effective clinician-patient interactions that can, in turn, affect medical effectiveness and health outcomes. Language fluency and literacy are also important considerations in the development of health promotion materials. Materials must be available in Spanish, be culturally sensitive to the heterogeneity of various Latino groups, and consider varying levels of education and literacy.

One of the remedial measures used to address language differences between the health care delivery system and the patient is the translator. However, the triangular interaction that results from the use of translators inevitably leads to gaps in clinician-patient communication (Carrasquillo et al. 1999b; Pérez-Stable et al. 1997; Rivadeneyra et al. 2000). Often, because of the lack of availability of professional medical interpreters, family members are used in this capacity, which can lead to problems. For example, Latino women may be reluctant to reveal personal problems when children are present, and overprotective family members also may censor critical medical information that they feel is unimportant.

Immigrants' experiences with medical practices in their native countries affect their expectations of care provided in the United States. American medical procedures may be very different from those practiced in other countries; therefore, thorough explanations and confirmation that the patient has understood are necessary. Lack of familiarity with the bureaucratic complexities of obtaining health care is especially critical in the current medical environment.

Access to Care

Latinos make up approximately 12% of the United States population, yet they constitute nearly one-fourth of the uninsured in this country (National Center for Health Statistics 2000). Nearly 4 in 10 Latinos are uninsured, reflecting the highest rates of any ethnic group in the United States. The percentage of uninsured Latinos varies by subgroup, from 21% for Cubans and Puerto Ricans to 38% for Mexicans and 42% for Central Americans (National Center for Health Statistics 2000). According to BRFSS data for 1999, 17.6% of the Latinos compared with 8.1% of the whites reported an inability to see a doctor in the last 12 months because of cost (Division of Adult and Community Health, National Center for Chronic Disease Prevention and Health Promotion et al. 2000).

It is not surprising that Latinos have the worst health insurance coverage of any ethnic group in the United States because of their low median income and tendency to be employed in lower-status occupations, which often do not offer benefits. In fact, most uninsured Latinos (87%) come from working families (National Center for Health Statistics 2000). Despite recent economic prosperity, Latinos disproportionately accounted for 36.4% of the growth in the number of uninsured in this country (Carrasquillo et al. 1999a). A study of the effects of acculturation on health care seeking in Mexican Americans (Solis et al. 1990) found that lower acculturation levels were associated with lower use of outpatient services for physical or emotional problems. Even for patients with Medicaid, when controlling for need, less acculturated patients used inpatient services four times less than did more acculturated patients.

According to 1998 data, the proportion of Latina women receiving no or late prenatal care was more than twice that of white women (6.3% vs. 2.4%) (Ventura et al. 2000). In 1992, only 62%–67% of Mexican, Puerto Rican, and Central American pregnant women received early prenatal care compared with 84%–88% of white and Cuban pregnant women.

CONCLUSIONS

Compared with other ethnic groups, Latinos tend to be relatively healthier, as evidenced by traditional indicators of morbidity and mortality. However, a significant variation in outcomes is associated with national origin and level of acculturation, and more data by subgroups are needed. Despite epidemiologic data that portray Latinos as relatively healthy, the self-perceived health status of Latinos may be quite different. According to 1998 NHIS data, Latinos were more likely to report poor or fair health than were whites (13.1% vs. 8.2%) (National Center for Health Statistics 2000).

The effects of acculturation and educational differences on health outcomes continue to be areas for further research. Socioeconomic and educational differences among Latinos and the effect of these factors on health and illness need to be better understood in the interface between the Latino patient and the health care system. Health care professionals need to understand culture-specific attitudes and behaviors and how they influence the processes of self-care, medical care, and follow-up.

Several structural factors, such as lack of insurance, lack of health care centers located in minority communities, reliance on public health systems (which typically means longer waits to schedule and see physicians), and a general lack of linguistically and culturally competent care, limit access to care for Latinos. In California, Latinos compose 31% of the population, yet only 4% of the physicians are Latino (Dower et al. 2001). More Latino health care providers need to be trained in all specialties of medicine, in the nursing professions, and in mental health as one mechanism by which to increase access to care.

REFERENCES

American Psychiatric Association: Diagnostic and Statistical Manual of Mental Disorders, 4th Edition, Text Revision. Washington, DC, American Psychiatric Association, 2000

Blackhall LJ, Murphy ST, Frank G, et al: Ethnicity and attitudes toward patient autonomy. JAMA 274:820–825, 1995

Canto MT, Chu KC: Annual cancer incidence rates for Hispanics in the United States. Cancer 88:2642–2652, 2000

Carrasquillo O, Himmelstein DU, Woolhandler S, et al: Going bare: trends in health insurance coverage, 1989 through 1996. Am J Public Health 89:36–42, 1999a [published erratum appears in Am J Public Health 89:256, 1999]

Carrasquillo O, Orav EJ, Brennan TA, et al: Impact of language barriers on patient satisfaction in an emergency department. J Gen Intern Med 14:82–87, 1999b

Castillo R, Waitzkin H, Ramirez Y, et al: Somatization in primary care, with a focus on immigrants and refugees. Arch Fam Med 4:637–646, 1995

Centers for Disease Control: HIV/AIDS Surveillance Report. January 1991, pp 1–22

Centers for Disease Control and Prevention: Cigarette smoking among adults—United States, 1997. MMWR Morb Mortal Wkly Rep 48:993–996, 1999

Centers for Disease Control and Prevention: Levels of diabetes-related preventive care practices—United States, 1997–1999. MMWR Morb Mortal Wkly Rep 49:954–958, 2000a

Centers for Disease Control and Prevention: Prevalence of leisure-time and occupational physical activity among employed adults—United States, 1990. MMWR Morb Mortal Wkly Rep 49:420–424, 2000b

Centers for Disease Control and Prevention: Surveillance for Selected Tobacco-Use Behaviors—United States, 1990–1995. Atlanta, GA, Tobacco Information and Prevention Source (TIPS), National Center for Chronic Disease Prevention and Health Promotion, Centers for Disease Control and Prevention, 2000c. Available at: http://www.cdc.gov/tobacco/research_data/adults_prev/tab_3.htm

Division of Adult and Community Health, National Center for Chronic Disease Prevention and Health Promotion, Centers for Disease Control and Prevention: Behavioral Risk Factor Surveillance System Online Prevalence Data, 1995–1999. Available at: http://apps.nccd.cdc.gov/brfss/index.asp

Division of HIV/AIDS Prevention, National Center for HIV, STD, and TB Prevention, Centers for Disease Control and Prevention: HIV/AIDS Surveillance by Race/Ethnicity (L238 slide series through 1999, slide 2 of 12), July 2000. Available at: http://www.cdc.gov/hiv/graphics/images/l238/l238-2.htm

Dower C, McRee T, Grumbach K, et al: The Practice of Medicine in California: A Profile of the Physician Workforce. San Francisco, CA, California Workforce Initiative at the UCSF Center for the Health Professions, February 2001

Flegal KM, Ezzati TM, Harris MI, et al: Prevalence of diabetes in Mexican Americans, Cubans, and Puerto Ricans from the Hispanic Health and Nutrition Examination Survey, 1982–1984. Diabetes Care 14:628–638, 1991

Haffner SM, Knapp JA, Hazuda HP, et al: Dietary intakes of macronutrients among Mexican Americans and Anglo Americans: the San Antonio heart study. Am J Clin Nutr 42:1266–1275, 1985

Harris MI, Flegal KM, Cowie CC, et al: Prevalence of diabetes, impaired fasting glucose, and impaired glucose tolerance in U.S. adults. The Third National Health and Nutrition Examination Survey, 1988–1994. Diabetes Care 21:518–524, 1998a

Harris MI, Klein R, Cowie CC, et al: Is the risk of diabetic retinopathy greater in non-Hispanic blacks and Mexican Americans than in non-Hispanic whites with type 2 diabetes? A U.S. population study. Diabetes Care 21:1230–1235, 1998b

Lavery LA, van Houtum WH, Ashry HR, et al: Diabetes-related lower-extremity amputations disproportionately affect blacks and Mexican Americans. South Med J 92:593–599, 1999

Marín G, Pérez-Stable EJ: Effectiveness of disseminating culturally appropriate smoking-cessation information: *Programa Latino Para Dejar de Fumar* (monograph). J Natl Cancer Inst 18:155–164, 1995

Marín G, Sabogal F, Marín BV, et al: Development of a short acculturation scale for Hispanics. Hispanic Journal of Behavioral Sciences 9:183–205, 1987

Marín G, Pérez-Stable EJ, Marín BV: Cigarette smoking among San Francisco Hispanics: the role of acculturation and gender. Am J Public Health 79:196–198, 1989

Marín G, Marín BV, Pérez-Stable EJ, et al: Cultural differences among Hispanics and non-Hispanic white smokers: attitudes and expectancies. Hispanic Journal of Behavioral Sciences 12:422–436, 1990

Mokdad AH, Ford ES, Bowman BA, et al: Diabetes trends in the U.S.: 1990–1998. Diabetes Care 23:1278–1283, 2000

Murphy SL: Deaths: final data for 1998. Natl Vital Stat Rep 48:1–20, 2000

National Center for Health Statistics: Health, United States, 2000, With Adolescent Health Chartbook. Hyattsville, MD, National Center for Health Statistics, 2000

Neff N: Empacho, in Folk medicine in Hispanics in the Southwestern United States (Module VII of Health Status and Determinants of Health of Hispanic Populations [online course]). Houston, TX, Baylor College of Medicine, Department of Community Medicine, 1996. Available at: http://riceinfo.rice.edu/projects/ HispanicHealth/Courses/mod7/empacho.html

Otero-Sabogal R, Sabogal F, Pérez-Stable EJ, et al: Dietary practices, alcohol consumption, and smoking behavior: ethnic, sex, and acculturation differences. J Natl Cancer Inst Monogr 18:73–82, 1995

Pachter LM: Culture and clinical care. JAMA 271:690–694, 1994

Pavlik VN, Hyman DJ, Vallbona C: Hypertension control in multi-ethnic primary care clinics. J Hum Hypertens 10 (suppl 3):S19–S23, 1996

Pérez-Stable EJ, Marín BV, Marín G, et al: Apparent underreporting of cigarette consumption among Mexican American smokers. Am J Public Health 80:1057–1061, 1990a

Pérez-Stable EJ, Marín G, Marín BV, et al: Depressive symptoms and cigarette smoking among Latinos in San Francisco. Am J Public Health 80:1500–1502, 1990b

Pérez-Stable EJ, Marín G, Marín BV, et al: Misclassification of smoking status by self-reported cigarette consumption. American Review of Respiratory Disease 145:53–57, 1992a

Pérez-Stable EJ, Sabogal F, Otero-Sabogal R, et al: Misconceptions about cancer among Latinos and Anglos. JAMA 268:3219–3223, 1992b

Pérez-Stable EJ, Benowitz NL, Marín G: Is serum cotinine a better measure of cigarette smoking than self-report? Prev Med 24:171–179, 1995

Pérez-Stable EJ, Nápoles-Springer A, Miramontes JM: The effect of ethnicity and language on medical outcomes of patients with hypertension or diabetes. Med Care 35:1212–1219, 1997

Pérez-Stable EJ, Marín G, Posner SF: Ethnic comparison of attitudes and beliefs about cigarette smoking. J Gen Intern Med 13:167–174, 1998

Pugh JA: Diabetic nephropathy and end-stage renal disease in Mexican Americans. Blood Purif 14:286–292, 1996

Ries LA, Wingo PA, Miller DS, et al: The annual report to the nation on the status of cancer, 1973–1997, with a special section on colorectal cancer (supplemental materials). Cancer 88:2398–2424, 2000

Rivadeneyra R, Elderkin-Thompson V, Silver RC, et al: Patient centeredness in medical encounters requiring an interpreter. Am J Med 108:470-474, 2000

Solis JM, Marks G, Garcia M, et al: Acculturation, access to care, and use of preventive services by Hispanics: findings from HHANES 1982–84. Am J Public Health 80 (suppl):11–19, 1990

Sundquist J, Winkleby M: Country of birth, acculturation status and abdominal obesity in a national sample of Mexican-American women and men. Int J Epidemiol 29:470–477, 2000

Triandis HC, Marín G, Lisansky J, et al: *Simpatia* as a cultural script of Hispanics. J Pers Soc Psychol 47:1363–1375, 1984

U.S. Department of Health and Human Services: Tobacco Use Among U.S. Racial/Ethnic Minority Groups—African Americans, American Indians and Alaska Natives, Asian Americans and Pacific Islanders, and Hispanics: A Report of the Surgeon General. Atlanta, GA, Centers for Disease Control and Prevention, National Center for Chronic Disease Prevention and Health Promotion, Office on Smoking and Health, 1998

Ventura SJ, Martin JA, Curtin SC, et al: Births: final data for 1998. Natl Vital Stat Rep 48:1–100, 2000

Wells AJ, English PB, Posner SF, et al: Misclassification rates for current smokers misclassified as nonsmokers. Am J Public Health 88:1503–1509, 1998

Winkleby MA, Kraemer HC, Ahn DK, et al: Ethnic and socioeconomic differences in cardiovascular disease risk factors: findings for women from the Third National Health and Nutrition Examination Survey, 1988–1994. JAMA 280:356–362, 1998

Zambrana RE, Breen N, Fox SA, et al: Use of cancer screening practices by Hispanic women: analyses by subgroup. Prev Med 29 (6 Pt 1):466–477, 1999

CHAPTER 3

Assessment and Treatment
of the Latino Patient

Ernestina Carrillo, M.S.W.

A COMPREHENSIVE AND ACCURATE evaluation of the Latino psychiatric patient requires that clinicians take into account information beyond what
is usually considered necessary in a conventional psychiatric intake. It is insuf-
ficient to concentrate solely on recent symptoms and circumstances when
reaching diagnostic and treatment conclusions. Latinos in the United States
are a diverse population, who are often influenced by cultural, social, and political systems quite different from those of the mainstream American population.
Inquiry must be made about how these differing factors affect the patient's
behavior and psychiatric presentation. The challenge for clinicians working
with Latinos in psychiatric settings is to learn how to take the broad, general
information about Latino culture and to apply it to the circumstances of the
individual patient without making oversimplified, stereotypical assumptions.
In this chapter I provide background information about Latinos and practical
guidelines on how to use this information in the assessment of the Latino
patient.

ASSESSMENT OF LANGUAGE

The first step in the assessment of the Latino patient is to determine what language the person most effectively and accurately uses to communicate. Pre-

ciado and Henry (1997) have classified Latinos into four categories according to their language dominance: 1) monolingual English speakers, 2) English-dominant bilinguals, 3) Spanish-dominant bilinguals, and 4) monolingual Spanish speakers.

It is important for clinicians to evaluate language fluency and not depend solely on the reliability of self-report. Patients who at times identify themselves as bilingual may have a command of English that allows them to function in the work world, but it is not the language they speak socially or in which they experience the full realm of life. In treatment settings, they are able to make their basic needs known but cannot elaborate with the specific detail necessary for the psychiatric interview. During the mental status examination these patients raise particular issues, depending on their command of English, because they present as either sicker or more healthy than they actually are, as in the following case example:

> Mr. B is a 20-year-old Salvadoran male, who was hospitalized on an inpatient psychiatric unit. He identified himself as being bilingual. Upon evaluation by the Spanish-speaking nursing staff, the Spanish-speaking staff who saw him as hypomanic questioned why the English-speaking psychiatrist was planning to treat him with antidepressants. A case conference was held in which the doctor interviewed Mr. B in English. During the interview the patient spoke in slow, halting English; his affect was flat, and his thoughts were incomplete. His answers to questions were succinct, and he provided scant information. The psychiatrist's diagnostic impression was that Mr. Martinez was depressed, with a psychotic thought process. When the Spanish-speaking staff interviewed Mr. B in Spanish, there was a dramatic change in his presentation. He became expansive in his responses and was quite delusional and labile. He provided a complete history, including details of having witnessed his brother killed during the civil war in El Salvador. He was also able to disclose symptoms that had previously remained hidden. The diagnostic impression after the interview was conducted in Spanish was posttraumatic stress disorder (PTSD) and bipolar affective disorder.

During the interview Mr. B's poor command of English made him appear to be thought blocking and either evasive or forgetful. Once he switched to Spanish, he had less control over his symptoms, since his concentration was no longer directed toward speaking English, and a clearer clinical picture emerged. He also had a larger vocabulary available, enabling him to provide a more detailed history that helped to further clarify the diagnoses.

Patients who are bilingual often present an interesting therapeutic challenge because they switch between the use of English and Spanish during the psychiatric interview (Marcos and Urcuyo 1979). At times they move from their primary to their secondary language to avoid difficult memories, topics, or emotions. This may occur at a conscious or an unconscious level. As one Mexican patient eloquently stated when confronted with her use of English as an avoidance mechanism in therapy, "English is where I defend myself, Spanish is where I feel." A parallel sentiment was expressed by another patient, who stated, "English is how I forget, Spanish is how I remember and cry."

When patients shift language in the interview, it is useful for clinicians to continue speaking in the patient's primary language. This maintains an emotional connection to what is being said and encourages patients to revert to their primary language. Clinicians who are uncomfortable with their own fluency in Spanish are often so relieved when a patient begins to speak English that they fail to notice the loss of content that occurs when the languages are switched.

One of the initial steps in the psychiatric interview of Latino patients is clinicians' stating what their own fluency in Spanish is. Latino patients often assume that non-Latino providers do not speak Spanish, and they similarly assume that Latino providers are fluent in Spanish. Simple statements like, "I'm fluent in Spanish," "I understand Spanish better than I speak it," or "I understand Spanish better when it is spoken slowly" help to clarify the clinician's language abilities, and this clarification encourages patients to be open about their own English speaking skills. Whatever the language preference of the clinician, it is important that patients not be obligated for the sake of the clinician to speak in a language with which they are uncomfortable.

Interpreters are recommended in situations where clinicians and patients do not share a common language. The efficacy of interpreted sessions depends on whether interpreters have been trained to work in psychiatric settings and on whether clinicians have been trained in how to work with an interpreter. Interpreters who do not understand the psychiatric interview process normalize patients' responses and omit details they do not understand or that embarrass them (Hornberger et al. 1997; Poss and Rangel 1995).

The following guidelines are useful when conducting a session where an interpreter is used:

- Meet with the interpreter before the session to provide information about the important highlights of the case and the type of information that will be elicited during the interview.
- Emphasize to the patient that confidentiality will be maintained, even though a session is being interpreted. This is particularly important if the interpreter and the patient are of the same cultural background.
- During the interview, maintain eye contact with the patient, not the inter-

preter, and use nonverbal behaviors such as nodding or facial expression to communicate that what the patient is saying is being understood.

- Observe the patient's body language to help ascertain that the interpreter is reporting what the patient has said. If incongruencies are noted between what the interpreter reports and how the patient appears, ask for clarification with statements like "Tell me why you are crying" or "You look frightened—tell me about it."

When a professional interpreter is not available, it is inappropriate to ask clerical staff to conduct interpretations unless there is an understanding that this is part of their job descriptions and they have been trained as interpreters. It is inappropriate and unprofessional to ask janitorial staff to serve as interpreters.

In clinics where Spanish-speaking professional staff members are expected to interpret for their non-Spanish-speaking peers, adjustments in their caseloads need to be made to reflect this extra duty. Furthermore, clinicians who serve as interpreters are to be treated as partners in the treatment. Their clinical impressions and recommendations should be elicited and respected.

There are occasions when the only interpreter available is a family member. Good practice dictates that family members are not to be used as interpreters. However, the reality is that some clinics do not have Spanish-speaking providers or interpreters. The dilemma becomes whether to allow a family member to act as interpreter or to deny the service. If Spanish-speaking services are available at other times of the day or in other treatment locations, it is best to refer patients to those services.

In situations where a family member is the absolutely only interpreter available, the following considerations must be taken into account:

- Young children or adolescents should never be used as interpreters, even if this means the patient has to go home and return with an adult.
- When a family member or friend acts as an interpreter, there needs to be an acknowledgment that confidentiality will not be maintained.
- Family members and friends are not impartial in their interpretations: they will ask and repeat only what they want the clinician to know. In most instances the interpretations are more reflective of the interpreter's viewpoint than the patient's.
- Patients may avoid revealing sensitive information because they do not want people close to them knowing their business or because certain issues are a source of conflict and they do not want to discuss them in the presence of the person doing the interpreting.

ACCULTURATION

When working with a Latino patient, it is important to evaluate the person's level of acculturation. *Acculturation* has been defined as the loss of traditional cultural attitudes, values, beliefs, customs, and behaviors and the acceptance of new cultural traits (Baròn and Constantine 1997; Keefe and Padilla 1987). It is considered a multifaceted, ongoing process. Several scales for acculturation have been developed and refined through the years (Cuellar et al. 1980; Marín et al. 1987; Vega et al. 1994). Items measured typically include language preference, media language preference, ethnic identification, awareness and loyalty, and adherence to traditional Latino family values.

People move along the acculturation continuum at different rates in different spheres of cultural activity (Keefe and Padilla 1987). An immigrant may make rapid changes in certain areas, out of the need for survival—such as learning the language or the economic system—but may still maintain very traditional attitudes about gender roles within the family or may feel most comfortable within a social network composed primarily of other Latinos. Similarly, a Latino born in the United States may no longer speak Spanish and may appear to subscribe to the values of the mainstream society, but he or she may still retain a strong sense of family loyalty and obligation, in concert with Latino values.

Latinos who are recent immigrant are often monolingual Spanish-speaking, they tend to socialize primarily with persons of their own group, and they closely adhere to traditional Latino cultural values. Variations occur, depending on whether persons come to the United States from urban or rural areas, what their class status was in their country of origin, and what economic resources are available to them in this country. Stressors experienced by this group include isolation, discrimination, low socioeconomic status, depression related to the losses they have experienced, and anxiety due to culture shock.

Latino immigrants who have been in the United States for an extended period often find themselves in cultural transition as blending occurs between the old and new cultures. Families in this group tend to be susceptible to high degrees of stress and intergenerational conflict. Children and adolescents are able to learn English more easily than are adults, and they are eager to take on the new culture as a way of fitting in with their peers, whereas their parents strive to keep cultural values intact as a way of keeping the past alive. Similarly, roles become reversed in marital relationships: women may become the primary breadwinners, often because they have more employment opportunities than do men.

Individuals who are born in this country or who immigrated at an early age may feel proficient in aspects of both the Latino and the American culture. The truly adept individual is often described as being bicultural and as having the ability to choose between the best (or worst) of what the two cultures have to offer. However, because the two cultures are so different and often have conflicting expectations, individuals may at times find themselves feeling caught between two worlds. Being bicultural does not mean being bilingual; therefore, some Latinos in this group may lack proficiency in Spanish or not speak Spanish. This lack can separate the person from the rest of the family if there are monolingual Spanish-speaking relatives such as grandparents, aunts, or uncles. Issues confronting upwardly mobile Latinos include feeling frustrated or guilty because many of their family members still continue to live in substandard, poverty conditions. Latino professionals sometimes struggle against the possibility of being seen as *vendidos,* or sellouts, as they choose career paths that are not seen as being directly beneficial to the Latino community or that take them away from the families and neighborhoods (Manoleas and Carrillo 1991).

Finally, there are Latinos who have acculturated and assimilated to the extent that they no longer identify themselves as Latino. Usually these persons are unaffected by culture until they encounter relatives who are still Latino identified and who chastise them for forgetting their Latino roots. Even though these acculturated persons do not think of themselves as Latino, they may still experience racism or discrimination because they have a Spanish surname or brown skin. This often feels shameful, confusing, and/or disorienting to them. Finally, some people who pass as Caucasian sometimes live with the anxiety of being discovered to be Latino.

LATINO CULTURE

A number of characteristics are shared by Latino groups, including family structure, gender roles, religion, and value systems. Variations in traditional cultural norms result from differences dictated by region, class, and generational status. However, the most important variations are those resulting from individual or family preference (Bernal 1982; Canino and Canino 1993; Martinez 1988).

Family

The functions of the traditional Latino family include taking care of children and the elderly and providing financial and emotional support to family members. The well-being of the family supersedes that of the individual. Latino families traditionally extend across generational lines. Although, in the United

States, households are generally composed of nuclear families, the concept of extended family remains important: included in the matrix of those called upon in decision making and for emotional support are grandparents, aunts or uncles, and cousins.

Kinship is often extended to persons outside the family, and these relationships are considered as important as bloodlines. The system of incorporated relatives includes the *compadres,* the godparents of children at baptism or sponsors in important events such as weddings, communions, confirmation, or sweet-fifteen *(quinceañero)* celebrations. *Hijos de crianza* are children who have been formally or informally adopted and have grown up as part of a household. *Parientes* are persons a family feels an affinity with and designates as adopted cousins, aunts, or uncles. Sometimes these relationships are so embedded within the family life that a patient insists that these persons be included when a genogram is constructed.

In assessment of Latino families it is important to note that there has been a diminishing of traditional bonds within the culture. Divorce, working parents, lack of leisure time, urbanization, acculturation, and acquisition of American values have affected these traditions (Canino and Canino 1993). However, clinicians may find that in times of crisis, such as during an illness, families often come together in support of the patient. Therefore, it is important to discover who these potential supports are and to evaluate how they can be integrated into treatment.

Immigration is disruptive to the traditional family structure; thus it is important to assess its impact on the individual and family life cycle (Lee 1991). For example, it is important to inquire who was left behind in the native country and how these separations have affected the family or patient. Most immigrants tend to go to communities in the United States where other people from their home country reside and to build secondary families for themselves. It is of diagnostic concern when immigrant individuals fail to establish new familylike connections and instead remain completely isolated in this country. Similarly, it is of concern when a family becomes unable to cope and relinquishes the care of one of its members completely to the mental health system.

Family cohesiveness, respect, and loyalty are highly valued in the Latino culture. There is an edict against telling family business to strangers (as alluded to in the previous section of this chapter discussing interpreters). Thus, patients seeking mental health services may initially refrain from revealing family conflicts as stressors because they do not want to betray the family. Clinicians can demonstrate sensitivity to this issue by ensuring confidentiality and explaining to the patient why information is being sought and how it will be used.

The following case example illustrates the importance of family cultural values to this Latina, even though she was quite acculturated:

A young Latina attorney sought treatment with a presenting complaint that she felt alienated in the work setting and was considering leaving the profession, even though she enjoyed her work and becoming an attorney had been her lifelong dream. Initially she had enjoyed her job and the opportunities facing her, but she felt her career come to a standstill when she began to set limits around how much time she could spend on work-related social events outside work hours. Also, her co-workers labeled her a tightwad because she would not join them for expensive lunches. In time, people stopped issuing invitations and she began to feel as though she did not exist in the office.

Assessment of her circumstances revealed that she had little time or money available for socializing. Most weekends she returned to her hometown to give her mother respite in the care of elderly parents, and weekday evenings she took care of her nieces and nephew so that her sister could work. Even though the attorney earned a good income, her money was spent helping younger siblings with their educational expenses, and she also assisted with the medical bills of several other family members. In college, when she had sought treatment for similar issues, the therapist advised her to break her dependency on her "enmeshed family." In treatment this second time, she was able to set a more acceptable goal of finding a way to balance family obligations and personal needs. Eventually, she was able to learn how to allot time and money for herself while still remaining a support to her family.

Family Roles

Traditional Latino families are organized along hierarchical lines, with defined gender roles (Bernal and Flores-Ortiz 1982). Males are generally seen as heads of their households and as providing financial support and protection for their families. Women's roles are typically assigned to the home. Their duties include daily management of the household, child rearing, and providing emotional support to family members. Females are given less autonomy than are males and are encouraged to stay close to the home. Their virginity is closely guarded until marriage.

It is important to mention the concepts of *machismo* and *marianismo* in the discussion of gender roles. In the media and larger society a *macho* is described as a Latino male who is aggressive, sexually adventurous, a wife beater, and a substance abuser, whereas in the Latino culture the traditional definition of a *macho* is a male who protects and provides for his family. Similarly, Latinas are described as *marianiastas*—modest, submissive, self-sacrificing women (Gill and Vasquez 1996).

Clinicians who subscribe to these stereotypical views of Latino male and female roles will overlook or tolerate maladaptive, dangerous behavior in an effort to provide culturally sensitive interventions. If maladaptive or danger-ous behaviors are occurring within any Latino family, clinicians must provide immediate intervention to ensure the safety of family members. (See Chapter 12 for a model for working with the issue of domestic violence.

Traditional roles are undergoing tremendous changes, which have accel-erated as more Latinas work outside the home, gain higher education, and be-gin to demand more equality and autonomy within the family. Latino males are more involved with their families than in previous generations. They have more integral roles in the lives of their children and are no longer seen as dis-ciplinarians who are to be respected from a distance. For some Latino families these changing roles may be experienced as stressful if they continue to subscribe to traditional roles and behaviors as the ideal of how families "should be."

Intergenerational conflict is common in Latino families, where parents and children often have differing levels of acculturation (Bernal and Flores-Ortiz 1982) and, as noted previously, the values of the original culture and of the United States are in conflict. In Latino culture, children are taught to be respectful of their elders and loyal to the family, putting needs of family mem-bers first, whereas American mainstream culture promotes independence and competition. For example, in a traditional Latino family, children are expected to be seen but not heard, and questioning an adult is seen as disrespectful; in many American school settings, on the other hand, children who excel are those who can think critically and ask challenging questions, and competition is valued and encouraged.

Immigrant children often experience role confusion. Because they have more opportunities to learn English, they are often called upon to interact with the larger society for their parents. They provide translation, fill out applica-tions, handle business transactions, and so forth, yet upon return home they are expected to revert to their roles of quiet, obedient children. Skilled clini-cians will act as culture brokers, helping parents and children see the world through each other's eyes and teaching them to negotiate compromises that will enhance family relationships.

Religion

Catholicism remains the primary religion for most Latinos, even though Pentecostal groups are having a major influence in many Central and South American countries. With many Latinos, the church is seen as a pri-mary support system. Some people faithfully and regularly attend reli-gious services, whereas others attend only on special occasions; however, many incorporate some form of prayer into their daily lives.

Traditionally, Latinos are very spiritual; in the literature, they are some-times described as fatalistic, because they see their destinies resting solely in the hands of God. They may feel that the only way to influence the course of their future is through prayer or other expressions of faith, such as lighting candles, constructing altars, or making promises and bargains with saints.

When in psychiatric distress, Latinos may interpret their symptoms as a deserved punishment for sins they have committed. In clinical intervention, Organista and Dwyer (1996) described incorporating people's spiritual beliefs and supports into the treatment. These therapists reinforce churchgoing and prayer as appropriate solutions for problems but also challenge these activities as not being enough to solve problems and to achieve symptom relief. They reframe spiritual and cultural beliefs such as *"si Dios quiere"* (if God so wishes) to *"ayudate, para que Dios te ayude"* (God helps those who help themselves).

It is important to help reengage people who have previously found solace in religion with this important source of support. Priests and other spiritual leaders are often quite willing to become partners in the treatment. Religious beliefs may also become useful tools in treatment; for example, very religious patients can sometimes control their suicide impulses because they see suicide as a sin against God.

ENGAGEMENT IN TREATMENT

The initial contact between clinician and patient is crucial in determining whether a Latino patient stays in treatment. Respect is an important cultural value that transcends all relationships that Latinos have; thus it becomes an important element in treatment. Respect can be conveyed simply by offering a handshake or making inquiry into the person's general well-being. When addressing the patient, it is important to use formal language—for example, use the formal "you," *usted,* rather than the familiar "you," *tù.* Also avoid overfamiliarity, such as using first names in greetings, particularly with older people.

It is also important to understand that Latino patients often try to form personal relationships with their treatment providers. They may ask personal questions, invite the clinician to family functions, or bring gifts of gratitude. It is therefore important for clinicians to educate patients about the bound-aries of the relationship, explaining both agency policy and professional ethics and why it is not therapeutic for professional relationships to become personal relationships. Most patients will respect and honor these restrictions.

Some self-disclosure by the clinician helps to develop the relationship.

Appropriate self-disclosure includes discussing one's area of expertise and professional credentials. A question commonly asked of Latino clinicians by their Latino patients is what their country of origin is; non-Latino patients who speak Spanish are often asked where they learned the language. Information shared about oneself needs to be very brief: for example, a clinician may want to share that his or her background is Puerto Rican, but it is not necessary to explain one's history in this country. A clinician who is asked a question that is too personal should not feel compelled to answer it and needs to redirect the patient to the purpose of the interview.

Reciprocity and showing one's appreciation is also an important cultural value; thus it is common for patients to bring their treatment providers gifts in gratitude for services provided. Good judgment must be used by clinicians as to whether to accept a gift. The acceptance of food or inexpensive tokens may be therapeutic to the relationship, but expensive or inappropriate gifts must be returned. An example: when a female client gave me a nightgown as a wedding gift, it was returned with a careful explanation of why it could not be accepted. The patient took the gift back, but the next week she returned with the gift of a dishtowel, which was graciously accepted, as it was very important to the client to acknowledge this important event in the therapist's life.

Finally, in engaging the patient, it is important to understand how Latino patients relate to their therapists, particularly to doctors. In Latino culture, there is great respect for doctors. Elderly women often dress up as if going to church when they have medical appointments, and there is great pride in families in which one of its members is a doctor or other health professional.

Latino patients have a tendency to address anyone who provides them with treatment as "doctor." Clinicians must therefore clarify their scope of practice—particularly mental health providers who have doctoral degrees. Latino patients are inclined to have loyalty to the individual doctor or clinician rather than to the institution where the person practices. It is difficult for patients to understand the transfer of their case to another clinician; they often experience it as a personal rejection.

One of the ways that Latino patients demonstrate respect toward doctors is by not disagreeing or asking questions. While in the office they outwardly agree with whatever the doctor says, even if they are in disagreement and have no intention of following the treatment recommendations; similarly, they often do not ask questions to clarify what they do not understand. Clinicians must therefore anticipate what the areas of question or disagreement may be and address these issues directly.

There is great stigma against mental illness in Latino culture, but at the same time there tends to be a great degree of tolerance for pathology. In psychiatric assessment, direct questions about whether any family members have had a mental illness usually yields "no" as an answer, but when the question is reframed in terms of symptoms, the clinician may learn that various family members have histories of isolative or erratic behavior or have died under circumstances that may be indicative of suicide. Because of the stigma related to mental illness, families may perceive accepting mental health services as a failure of the family system to take care of its own members; they may also feel shame. Further, as previously mentioned, they may fear that the treatment of one of its members will expose the privacy of the family.

As you will read in the following chapters in this book, many immigrant families come from countries where the mental health systems are very different from those in the United States. In many Latin American countries, mental health treatment is reserved for the most severely ill.

The following guidelines will enhance the engagement of these patients in treatment:

- Evaluate what the patient understands about psychiatric treatment and what his or her expectations are.
- Provide education about the psychiatric evaluation and intervention process.
- If treatment is involuntary, ensure that patients understand their rights and the legal issues involved.
- Include the patient's family in the treatment process.
- Practice creativity and flexibility. Both the treatment provider and the agency should do this. For example, treatment providers can act as case managers to obtain services for their patients; and agencies can provide evening hours for working people to come to the clinic, since most poor immigrants do not have jobs with the flexibility to let them attend medical appointments during the workday.

MENTAL STATUS EXAMINATION AND PSYCHIATRIC DIAGNOSES

A number of societal and cultural factors make the psychiatric diagnoses of Latinos difficult (Flaskerud and Hu 1992; Rogler 1993). Latinos in the United States often live under stressful life conditions, which may include poverty, low occupational status, lack of proficiency in English, and undocumented legal status. Immigration and associated problems such as separation from family members, the effects of having witnessed brutal acts of war and violence, having lived under political oppression, or having experienced torture can exacerbate these social problems (Carrillo 1991). In working with Latino psychiatric patients, it is at times difficult to distinguish appropriate reactions to overwhelming life stressors from reactions that are beyond the realm of normal grief or response (López 1991). In making psychiatric diagnoses it is important to use the criteria set forth in DSM-IV (American Psychiatric Association 1994) while at the same time taking into consideration cultural responses to stress and cultural expression of symptoms. As with any patient, a detailed history and, when available, collateral information help to clarify the diagnoses. The specificity of a detailed history helps the clinician get beyond the description Latinos often use as to what is going on with them as being merely *nervios,* or "nerves," a term that is used to encompass symptoms ranging from everyday blues to severe psychotic disorders (López 1991).

For example, clinicians sometimes have difficulty determining whether strong religious thinking in a patient can be termed as hyperreligious or whether it is within the realm of being culturally appropriate. Clarification is further complicated because some patients and their families see their symptoms as either a gift from God or a deserved punishment and therefore resist intervention.

López (1991) suggested that diagnoses and the need for intervention can be clarified if the symptoms are assessed from the following perspectives:

- Is the religious preoccupation a new or different behavior for the patient?
- Has it increased or decreased in expression?
- Is it interfering with the patient's daily functioning?
- Do people who know the patient think that the behavior has become excessive?
- Has the religious preoccupation endangered the patient's judgment or health?

Similarly, when diagnosing other psychiatric disorders, López (1991) recommended that the following points be considered:

- Consider depression in the presence of unexplained, persistent somatic complaints.
- Alcohol may be a contributing factor to many mood disorders.
- Many Latino immigrants come from countries where paranoia serves a functional role in the individual's life, since it is difficult to know who can or cannot be trusted; thus paranoid symptoms must be evaluated in a historical context.
- In evaluating symptoms, consideration must be given to the difficulties of

adjusting to a new environment where the person does not speak the language or understand the culture or may possibly have undocumented immigration status. All of these stressors can make a person guarded and suspicious.

- PTSD is difficult to diagnose because patients are often skilled at suppressing their painful memories and symptoms. Nightmares, unexplained somatic distress, new and unexplained antisocial behavior, intense fear and paranoia, and/or nightmares are often indicative of PTSD.

Another complicating factor in diagnoses of psychiatric disorders is that Latinos tend to seek treatment in primary care settings, where their psychiatric diagnoses are often missed or misdiagnosed (Pérez-Stable et al. 1990). There is a tendency in Latino culture to express psychological distress through physical symptoms (to somatize) (Escobar 1987). These symptoms include headaches, gastric distress, and general malaise and often have no discernible organic etiology. Patients with these types of symptoms can be quite frustrating to the medical provider, and they often are labeled as complainers rather than being given a mental health referral.

Patients with somatic distress who are seen by psychiatrists or therapists often feel frustrated because they do not see these clinicians as having the ability to cure their physical discomfort. The following guidelines are helpful in working with patients who present their symptoms in somatic form:

- Validate their physical concerns before embarking on an assessment of psychiatric symptoms.
- Inquire how long the symptoms have been present, how severe the pain is, what the patient thinks is causing the discomfort, and what remedies have been tried.
- In exploring psychological issues, explain the connection between one's physical and mental well-being.

CONCLUSIONS

It is important to consider the role played in the clinical presentation by the stress of being a Latino in the United States. As mentioned several times in this chapter and others, Latinos in the United States are by and large a poor population who live in substandard housing and who work long hours at low-paying jobs. For many of these people, despair is a chronic life condition. Along with poverty, institutional racism is another assaultive factor that affects the daily lives of Latinos. It feels disheartening to continuously see legislation introduced and passed that infringes on the group's basic rights. This despair is passed on generationally and results in new sets of social problems.

Immigrants have additional levels of stress. Many are forced to immigrate by the political situations in their homelands or by poor economic conditions. They have often left important family members behind and miss them tremendously. People who come from war-torn countries may experience delayed grief reactions for persons who died years ago but whom they have not had the opportunity to mourn. Some immigrants are unable to adjust to life in the United States because their intention is to return to their country of origin whenever the political or economic situation improves; as a result, their lives are in limbo. Some people are forced to immigrate against their will—for example, children, adolescents, and elderly persons—which creates family conflict. Professionals who immigrate often experience a loss of status because they are unable to practice their professions in the United States. For example, many Nicaraguan physicians who left their country during the revolution now earn their living in this country working as orderlies, laboratory technicians, or janitors in hospitals across the United States. Finally, it must be recognized that a large number of Latino immigrants have undocumented status and live in continuous fear of being caught and deported. This group is particularly vulnerable to being exploited in the society.

The field of Latino mental health has continued to expand during the past decades, but there is still much that we do not know and questions that still need to be asked in order to advance its practice. According to Roberts (1994), these questions include the following:

- What is the prevalence, incidence, and natural history of mental disorders in Latinos?
- What are the consequences of these clinical disorders?
- What are the joint effects of minority status, ethnic group, culture, and social class on psychiatric risk?

In this chapter the focus has been on practical guidelines in the engagement and assessment of Latino patients in psychiatric settings rather than on specific diagnostic categories or treatment modalities. In the next chapters of the book, Latinos are discussed in the context of their specific countries of origin, and further refinement is added to the generalities offered in this chapter.

REFERENCES

American Psychiatric Association: Diagnostic and Statistical Manual of Mental Disorders, 4th Edition. Washington, DC, American Psychiatric Association, 1994

Baròn A, Constantine MG: A conceptual framework for conducting psychotherapy with Mexican-American college students (Chapter 7), in Psychological Interventions and Research With Latino Populations. Edited by Garcìa JG, Zea MC. Boston, MA, Allyn & Bacon, 1997

Bernal G: Cuban families (Chapter 9), in Ethnicity and Family Therapy. Edited by McGoldrick M, Pearce JK, Giordano J. New York, Guilford, 1982

Bernal G, Flores-Ortiz Y: Latino families in therapy: engagement and evaluation. J Marital Fam Ther 8:357–365, 1982

Canino IA, Canino GJ: Psychiatric care of Puerto Ricans, in Culture, Ethnicity and Mental Illness. Edited by Gaw AC. Washington DC, American Psychiatric Press, 1993, pp 467–499

Carrillo E: Engaging the immigrant or refugee patient in treatment, in Immigrants and Refugees: A Handbook of Clinical Care. Edited by López AG, Lee E, Farr F. San Francisco, CA, University of California San Francisco School of Medicine, 1991

Cuellar I, Harris LC, Jasso R: An acculturation scale for Mexican-American normal and clinical populations. Hispanic Journal of Behavioral Sciences 2:199–217, 1980

Escobar JI: Cross-cultural aspects of the somatization trait. Hospital and Community Psychiatry 38:174–180, 1987

Farr F: A cultural framework explanatory model of illness, in Immigrants and Refugees: A Handbook of Clinical Care. Edited by López AG, Lee E, Farr F. San Francisco, CA, University of California San Francisco School of Medicine, 1991

Flaskerud JH, Hu L: Relationship of ethnicity to psychiatric diagnosis. J Nerv Ment Dis 180:296–303, 1992

Gil RM, Vasquez CI: The Maria Paradox: How Latinas Can Merge Old World Traditions With New World Self-Esteem. New York, GP Putnam's Sons, 1996

Hornberger J, Itakura H, Wilson SR: Bridging language and cultural barriers between physicians and patients. Public Health Rep 112(5):410–417, 1997

Keefe SE, Padilla AK: Chicano Ethnicity. Albuquerque, NM, University of New Mexico Press, 1987

Lee E: Assessment and evaluation of immigrant and refugee families, in Immigrants and Refugees: A Handbook of Clinical Care. Edited by López AG, Lee E, Farr F. San Francisco, CA, University of California San Francisco School of Medicine, 1991

López AG: Diagnostic issues and Latinos, in Immigrants and Refugees: A Handbook of Clinical Care. Edited by López AG, Lee E, Farr F. San Francisco, CA, University of California San Francisco School of Medicine, 1991

Manoleas P, Carrillo E: A culturally syntonic approach to the field education of Latino students. Journal of Social Work Education 27:135–144, 1991

Marcos LR, Urcuyo L: Dynamic psychotherapy with the bilingual patient. Am J Psychother 33:331–338, 1979

Marín G, Sabogal F, Marín BV, et al: Development of a short acculturation scale for Hispanics. Hispanic Journal of Behavioral Sciences 9:183–205, 1987

Martinez C: Mexican Americans, in Clinical Guidelines in Cross-Cultural Mental Health. Edited by Comas-Diaz L, Griffith EEH. New York, Wiley, 1988, pp 182–201

Organista KC, Dwyer EV: Clinical case management and cognitive-behavioral therapy: integrated psychosocial services for depressed Latino primary care patients (Chapter 5), in The Cross-Cultural Practice of Clinical Case Management in Mental Health. Edited by Manoleas P. Binghamton, NY, The Haworth Press, 1996

Pérez-Stable E, Miranda J, Muñoz R, et al: Depression in medical outpatients: underrecognition and misdiagnosis. Arch Intern Med 150:1083–1088, 1990

Poss JE, Rangel R: Working effectively with interpreters in the primary care setting. Nurs Pract 20:43–47, 1995

Preciado J, Henry M: Linguistic barriers in health education and services (Chapter 13), in Psychological Interventions and Research With Latino Populations. Edited by Garcìa JG, Zea MC. Boston, MA, Allyn & Bacon, 1997

Roberts RE: Research on the mental health of Mexican origin children and adolescents, in Latino Mental Health: Current Research and Policy Perspectives (monograph). Edited by Telles C, Karno M. Los Angeles, CA, National Institute of Mental Health and Neuropsychiatric Institute, University of California Los Angeles, 1994

Rogler LH: Culturally sensitive psychiatric diagnosis: a framework for research. J Nerv Ment Dis 181:401–408, 1993

Vega W, Zimmerman RS, Warheit GH: The role of cultural factors in mental health problems of Hispanic adolescents, in Latino Mental Health: Current Research and Policy Perspectives (monograph). Edited by Telles C, Karno M. Los Angeles, CA, National Institute of Mental Health and Neuropsychiatric Institute, University of California Los Angeles, 1994

PART II

Latino Peoples:
Cultural and Psychiatric Issues

CHAPTER 4

Colombians

Ramon A. Rojano, M.D., M.P.H.

LOCATED IN THE NORTHWEST corner of South America, Colombia is a beautiful and geographically diverse country with coasts in both the Atlantic and Pacific oceans. It borders five countries: Panama on the northwest, Venezuela on the northeast, Ecuador and Peru on the south, and Brazil on the southeast. The country's area of 440,381 square miles equals the combined areas of Spain, Portugal, and France. Colombia lies above the equator, and the climate varies significantly from one region to another, given the complexity and richness of its land and the various altitude levels. The country has high mountains where snow is perpetual, its interior has plateaus of temperate climate, and on its coasts the temperature is the same as that of the Caribbean islands. The topography is dominated by three Andean ranges that cross the country from southwest to northeast, originating at the Macizo Colombiano, where Colombia's two main rivers begin: the Magdalena and the Cauca (Embassy of the Republic of Colombia to the United States 2001; World Book Inc. 2001).

Colombia is divided into five main geographical regions:

- The Andean region, where most of the population is concentrated
- The Caribbean region, to the north, which features a very warm climate year round and beautiful beaches
- The Pacific region, to the west, which is covered by tropical rain forests and exuberant vegetation

- The Eastern Plains region, a mainly agricultural area and one of the richest in the country after the discovery of the Cano Limon oil field (1986) and the Cusiana and Cupiagua oil fields (1991)
- The Amazon region, to the southeast, covered by tropical rain forests and jungles

Colombia's territories also encompass two pieces of the Caribbean paradise, the islands of San Andres and Providence (Embassy of the Republic of Colombia to the United States 2001; U.S. Department of State 2000).

Colombia's history is fascinating, and is intense as well. Precolonial Colombia was the home of powerful Indian cultures. The first Spanish settlements were established in 1509, and after the founding of Santa Fe de Bogota, in 1538, the viceroyalty of Nueva Granada was established. A new ethnicity—the *criolos*, or *mestizos*—was developed out of the mix of Indians, Europeans, and Africans. Almost three centuries later the national independence movement, led by Simon Bolivar, was successful, and the Spaniards were defeated. In 1819, the independent republic of La Gran Colombia was declared, including then Colombia, Ecuador, Panama, and Venezuela. In 1830, Venezuela and Ecuador became separate nations, and many years later, in 1903, Panama also became independent. Since its inception, Colombia has been almost uninterruptedly a democratic country, which elects a president every 4 years. In its current geopolitical structure, Colombia is divided into 32 departments (similar to states) with governors elected directly by the citizens (Embassy of the Republic of Colombia to the United States 2001).

DEMOGRAPHICS

With an estimated population of 37,577,000 inhabitants, Colombia is the third most highly populated Spanish-speaking country in the world, with a growth rate that has steadily declined (from 2.3% in 1970 to 1.9% in 1990) (Departamento Administrativo Nacional de Estadistica 2001; Embassy of the Republic of Colombia to the United States 2001; U.S. Bureau of the Census 1993; U.S. Department of State 2000). In 1991, the population was distributed as follows: Andean region, 41%; Atlantic, 20%; Pacific, 16%; and District of Santa Fe de Bogota, 16% (Departamento Administrativo Nacional de Estadistica 2001). During the past 30 years, the age distribution has changed: individuals under 15 years of age accounted for 46.8% of the population in 1965, but only for 34% in 1993. Females, making up 50.8% of the population, slightly outnumbered males. The urban population increased from 42.1% in 1951 to 74% in 1993. With approximately 80 groups and 450 communities, the indigenous population was estimated in the 1993 census at approximately 1,106,499 individuals, living primarily in the Amazon, Orinoco, and Guajira regions and in the Andean Mountains (Departamento Administrativo Nacional de Estadistica 2001).

Although Colombia is a country rich in natural resources, many of its inhabitants are very poor. It is a nation of contrasts, with major social class differences. Although some are very wealthy, the majority of the population struggle to survive, and the middle class is almost nonexistent. In 1995, the average per capita gross income was approximately $1,210 per year (Inter-American Bank of Development 1999). Poverty is common in rural areas as well as in the periphery of major urban centers, where migrants from farms and small villages live in shanty towns, or *tugurios,* forming what have been described as suburban "belts of misery" (Pan American Health Organization 1994).

EDUCATION AND RELIGION

Colombia has enjoyed a hemisphere-wide reputation for intellectual achievement. Education is certainly one of the foremost values of a country where motivation for educational attainment is high. School participation has increased substantially in the past decades. Enrollment in preschool education increased from 15,365 children in 1978 to 1,034,182 in 1999. In elementary education, it increased from 3,608,859 children in 1978 to 5,162,260 in 1999. During the same period, the figures also increased for high school education, from 1,458,817 to 3,494,083 students (Departamento Administrativo Nacional de Estadistica 2001). Throughout the years, literacy has increased to 87% of the adult population, as reported in 1997 estimates. Nevertheless, even though primary education is free and compulsory from 6 to 14 years of age, approximately 10% of children do not attend school. It is believed by some that the 2.9% of Colombia's GNP and the 21% of the national budget that the government invests in education is not enough to appropriately reach out to and educate children living in very poor and distressed social environments (Pan American Health Organization 1999).

Roman Catholicism continues to be the most common religion, with a reported affiliation of about 90% of the population.

EMPLOYMENT

High unemployment rates have been constant in the past decades in Colombia. The situation worsened with a severe economic recession at the turn of the new century. According to the Departamento Administrativo Nacional de Estadistica (2001), the national unemployment rate as of February 2001 was 16.6%, and the underemployment rate was 30.9%. Unemployment tends to be lower in major capital cities and higher in rural areas. In regard to occupational distribution, a 1990 study showed that of 4,324,688 persons employed in seven metropolitan areas, 22% worked in community services, 21% in retail and business, and 20% in manufacturing (Departamento Administrativo Nacional de Estadistica 1990).

VIOLENCE

As a social phenomenon, *la violencia* has been a constant in the background of Colombia's history for about half of a century. Starting in the late 1940s, large-scale guerrilla activity and other chronic forms of violence have been a distressing reality that has altered the lives of many communities. Violence is also directly or indirectly responsible for the emigration of thousands of individuals to the United States and other countries. Since 1986, homicide has been the leading cause of death in Colombia, and its homicide rate of 86 per 100,000 is one of the highest in the world. In 1998, violent criminal attacks and homicide accounted for 45% of deaths in persons between 15 and 45 years of age. Homicide rates are extremely high in some cities, such as Antioquia (277/100,000 in 1991) and Valle (182/100,000 in 1991).

The Pan American Health Organization reported that, in 1995, there were a total of 1,450,845 years of potential life lost (YPLL) because of violent deaths, 67.4% (977,725) of which were due to homicide. In 1995, homicides were the leading cause of death for young Colombian males as well as the number-one cause of mortality and YPLL (67.4% of the total). In 1938, the homicide rate was 15 per 100,000 inhabitants; in the 1950s, despite the violence that marked this period, the rate was 55 per 100,000. In 1991, the rate peaked at 88 per 100,000 but then fell to 78 per 100,000 in 1994 and to 72 per 100,000 in 1995 (Europe World Book 2000; Pan American Health Organization 1999).

Colombia's three major cities, Santa Fe de Bogota, Medellin, and Cali, account for 64.5% of all homicides. This chronic situation not only has caused the displacement of farmers but also has prevented further development of many regions of the country, generated a new social underclass of dislocated people who migrate to the cities trying to survive, and caused major distress to children and families. In 2000, 315,384 individuals were reportedly dislocated because of violence (Grupo Temático de Desplazamiento 2000). The additional presence of drug trafficking and its associated terrorist activities has also aggravated the victimization of the population and has contributed to a decrease in the resources available for social investment (Europe World Book 2000; Pan American Health Organization 1999).

COLOMBIANS IN THE UNITED STATES

The Colombian population in the United States has continued to grow in the past few decades. According to Census Bureau estimates, 230,000 Colombians legally emigrated to the United States between 1981 and 1998 (124,000 in 1981–1990, 81,000 in 1991–1996, and 24,800 in 1997–1998) (U.S. Bureau of the Census 2000). Acquiring accurate data about the U.S. Colombian population has been a continuing challenge. U.S. Census Bureau data do not include nonresidents admitted for a temporary period, nor do they include undocumented immigrants or other migrants in transit. A large number of Colombians are here legally and temporarily with tourist and student visas. The Census Bureau estimated that between 1982 and 1996, approximately 62,000 Colombians overstayed in the United States without having the appropriate documentation (U.S. Bureau of the Census 1998).

According to the 1990 United States census (U.S. Bureau of the Census 1993), of the 378,726 Colombians living in the United States, 52.4% were female and 47.6% male. Foreign-born Colombians accounted for 74.2%; 25.8% were born in the United States. Colombians are the sixth largest Hispanic group in the United States (after Mexicans, Puerto Ricans, Cubans, Salvadorans, and Dominican Republicans), and the Colombian foreign-born population represents 3.6% of all foreign-born persons residing in the United States. The majority of immigrants (51.8%) entered the country between 1980 and 1990. Only 79,091, or 28% of the foreign-born, were naturalized citizens. Primary settlements of Colombians are New York (28.91%), Florida (23.3%), New Jersey (14.1%), California (19.6%), Texas (4.3%), and Illinois (2.6%) (U.S. Bureau of the Census 1993).

Among U.S. Colombians 25 years of age or older, 67.1% had completed at least a high school education. Sixteen percent had obtained at least a bachelor's degree, and 6.2% a master's or a doctoral degree. In 1990, there were 69,665 children enrolled in elementary or high school, and 45,161 individuals were attending college. The vast majority, 90.5%, were fluent in Spanish, and 53% reported that they did not speak English "very well." Among all Colombians, 32% were considered to be living in linguistically isolated households.

Technical and sales jobs were the most common occupations of Colombian immigrants (28%), followed by service-related jobs (21.6%) and managerial and professional jobs (17.1%). Of 88,617 families, 30% had one worker, 45% had two workers, and 19.6% had three or more workers. The unemployment rate was 8.4%. The median family income was $29,171, and the median per capita income was $11,150. Thirteen percent of families and 15.1% of individuals lived below the poverty level. Of 112,227 households, 30,067 (26.8%) were owner-occupied housing units (U.S. Bureau of the Census 1993).

HISTORY OF MIGRATION

According to the Colombian census, emigration exceeded 500,000 individuals in 1993. However, this number represents only half of the exodus, because much of the migration is done clandestinely (Pan American Health Organization 1999). Although Colombian migration to the United States started many years ago, it began to increase in the 1960s and peaked in the 1980s, when 124,000 Colombians were admitted into the United States (Heaton et al. 2000; U.S. Bureau of the Census 1999) (see Table 4–1).

Table 4–1. Colombian immigration

Period	Population (in thousands)
1961–1970	70.3
1971–1980	77.6
1981–1990	124.4
1988	10.3
1989	15.2
1990	24.2
1991	19.7
1992	13.2
1993	12.8
1994	10.8
1995	10.8
1996	14.3
Total	353.9

Source.   Heaton et al. 2000; U.S. Bureau of the Census 1999.

A survey conducted among Colombian immigrants in 1993 found the following reasons for migration: seeking a better job, seeking political refuge, escaping from a difficult family situation, looking for graduate or doctoral education, escaping from a violent environment, and searching for an international experience (Rojano 1993). More recently, exposure to higher levels of violence, experiences related to kidnappings or death threats, and frustration due to intensification of the political conflict are among the factors that have contributed to the massive interest in emigrating from Columbia (Forero 2001; Velez et al. 1997).

In the past, the fact that the vast majority of Colombians in the United States were not naturalized citizens was a factor that prevented them from participating actively in the American political process. Colombians were reluctant to seek U.S. citizenship because they did not want to lose their Colombian citizenship. However, this situation changed drastically in 1991 with the adoption of a new Colombian constitution that, among other provisions, allows for dual citizenship (Gaviria et al. 1991). Now, seeking naturalization has become a common trend. As a consequence, the level of political participation has increased to the point that Colombians in the United States have started to run for public office.

Cultural Patterns

The task of describing a unique psychological profile of Colombians is impossible because of the country's diversity in geography, ethnicity, and socioeconomic conditions. For example, in the Andean Mountains social behaviors tend to resemble those of other Andean countries, such as Peru or Bolivia; on the Caribbean coast, people exhibit cultural patterns similar to those of other Caribbean countries such as Cuba, Puerto Rico, or the Dominican Republic. Differences in cultural patterns are influenced, among other factors, by the type of regional *mestizajes,* or mixes, of people. These result from variations in local Indian tribes, differences in the type of Spaniards that settled in different regions, and the presence or absence of African heritage in a particular area, in combination with other factors such as social class differences, academic achievement, and differences between urban and rural environments (Gutierrez de Pineda 1975a, 1975b; Lopez et al. 1983).

Nevertheless, some shared cultural values are translated into frequent behaviors. Colombians, on the positive side, tend to be hard working, family oriented, resourceful, creative, patriotic, entrepreneurial, generous, witty, joyful, polite, self-reflective, and spiritual. On the other hand, shame, low self-esteem, guilt, and a tendency to foster classism can also be found. Various attempts have been made to study the Colombian culture, and descriptions of socioeconomic characteristics and cultural patterns of specific regional groups have been made.

The most important work is the vast research of anthropologist Virginia Gutierrez de Pinedo, who described four basic "cultural complexes": Andean-American (central region), Andean Neo-Hispanic (western region); Negroid (coasts and river basins), and Mountaineer (Antioquian region). In her two major books, Gutierrez (1975a, 1975b) described cultural patterns that were subsequently corroborated by many other studies in the description of the Colombian traditional family. These patterns tend to show a separation of male and female roles, with signs of behaviors that have been described as *machismo* and *marianismo* in other countries. In traditional families the tendency is for the father to assume the role of the provider and for the wife to serve as the emotional caretaker of the family. However, we need to be aware that these traditional patterns are rapidly changing in a country where women, who are playing a more active role in society, have not only massively joined the labor market in the last two decades, but also are now attaining higher education at a rate equal to or higher than that of males (Rojano 1985a, 1985b).

INCIDENCE OF MENTAL ILLNESS

In 1996, a large-scale nationwide mental health and substance abuse epidemiological study was conducted by researchers from the University of Antioquia and the University CES of Medellin. Funded by the Ministry of Health and working with a national team of more than 100 interviewers, the researchers interviewed a random sample of 15,046 individuals older than 12 years of age across the country, using the Clinical Diagnostic Inventory II questionnaire, which is based on the DSM-IV classification. This is the most comprehensive mental health study ever conducted in Colombia. The lifetime prevalence of diagnosable disorders was as follows: nicotine dependency, 28%; major depression, 19.3%; alcohol abuse and dependency (combined), 16.6%; posttraumatic stress disorder, 4.5%; somatization, 4.3%; generalized anxiety, 3.8%; and schizophrenia, 1.4%. The lifetime use of marijuana was 7.8% and of cocaine 2.5% (Torres and Montoya 1997). Suicide is also a public health problem; in 1995, a total of 58,830 suicides were reported in Columbia (Pan American Health Organization 1999).

RESOURCES IN MENTAL HEALTH

In 1994, Colombia had 35,640 physicians, an average of 9.4 physicians per 1,000 inhabitants. However, as reported by the Colombian Psychiatric Society, in 1996 the country had a population of more than 37 million and only approximately 700 psychiatrists, 1 per approximately 52,000 persons. Almost half are located in Santa Fe de Bogota, the capital, and jobs are available for them only in hospitals and other large institutions, not in small primary care clinics. Efforts to provide mental health training to primary care providers have been successful in Cali, where physicians and nurses have for years been involved in the treatment of mental illnesses and engaged in research as well. Nevertheless, all over the country, primary care physicians are very often confronted with many psychiatric clients without having the necessary training, experience, or resources to treat them appropriately.

Thirteen residency programs in psychiatry existed in 1996, with an enrollment of approximately 100 residents. Psychiatrists are organized primarily through the Colombian Psychiatric Society, which had approximately 500 members in 1996. The society produces a high-quality quarterly journal, *La Revista Colombiana de Psiquiatria*. The establishment of two psychiatric associations, the 250-member Colombian Association of Biological Psychiatry (1992) and the 75-member College of Neuropsychological Psychiatry (1996), may reflect a contemporary tendency of the profession toward biological psychiatry.

Since 1970, the number as well as the role of psychologists in Colombia has been substantially enhanced. Previously functioning primarily as an auxiliary of psychiatry, psychology has evolved during the last few decades, becoming the second leading profession in the mental health system and not only providing psychotherapeutic services but engaging in community work and scientific research as well. A study in 1983 found that approximately 4,500 psychologists had graduated in Colombia. In 1993, 16 pregraduate psychology programs and 8 graduate programs were available. In 1996, psychology masters' degrees were offered in the following areas: clinical psychology, health psychology, community psychology, and child psychology (Ardila 1993).

The vast majority of psychologists are concentrated in urban centers. A recent study (Ardila 1993) showed that 40.8% of psychologists work for governmental institutions, 58.1% work in private institutions, and 1.1% work independently. Clinical psychology is the preferred area of specialty (42.9%), followed by educational psychology (20.6%). Six percent of psychologists are dedicated to teaching. Psychologists are organized in more than a dozen associations throughout the country, the two most important being the Colombian Psychology Federation and the Colombian Society of Psychology. They are very active both professionally and academically, as shown by the 10 different psychological journals published and the approximately 15 annual national conventions held. Psychologists work with a variety of clinical approaches, of which psychodynamic and behavioral are the most popular.

As of 1996, more than 12,000 individuals had already completed their education in the existing 16 undergraduate social work programs of the country. Social workers in Colombia once served almost solely as providers of social assistance to impoverished individuals in hospitals and other urban institutions, but their role has expanded significantly in the past decade. Twelve graduate programs are now available, providing training in family interventions, community development, prevention, research, and program administration. Even though the majority of social workers are not engaged in the provision of psychotherapy, they play a major role in Colombia's mental health services delivery system. They use an ecosystem approach, linking clients with services, providing education and training to families, and organizing communities.

MENTAL HEALTH SYSTEM

With a few variations, the existing mental health system in Colombia follows the patterns of the existing general health care system, which is fairly new (U.S. Library of Congress 1998). A major overhaul of the old health care system stemmed from the new 1991 Constitution (Constitucion Politica de Colombia) and was legislated through "Law 100," or Ley 100, which passed in 1993 (Seguridad Social en Colombia 2001). With regard to health, the new Constitution's articles 48 and 49 declare that health is an inalienable right and guarantee access to the Social Security system to all Colombians (Gaviria et al. 1991). As stated, this Social Security system could be provided by the government and/or the private sector, opening the door for the establishment of public-private ventures. Previously, less than 20% of Colombians had guaranteed medical insurance. The rest of the nonpoor population had access to health care by paying in cash to private providers, and the poor had access to services through the old National Health Care System. This system was basically underfunded, and services were very limited. Law 100, legislated with the intention of increasing access to health services, introduced three major changes:

- Implementation of the Plan Obligatorio de Salud (POS; compulsory health plan) for all workers.
- Creation of the *empresas proveedoras de salud* (EPS), or health care providers, which are public and/or private organizations, agencies, or institutions that receive funding to provide health services.
- Creation of the System of Beneficiaries (SISBEN) to provide services to people who fall into classes I, II, or III of social status, status I being the poorest of the poor.

A massive campaign was launched to register all low-income Colombians in the SISBEN. Through all of these measures, a major and historic transformation of the Colombian health care system is under way. The current decentralized system consists of multiple private or public-private health care providers. The previously existing managed care companies became organized as health care providers (EPS) and/or started to offer supplemental plans for those with access only to the POS, which pays for limited services only. Within this new system, private practice has decreased substantially and in some specialties may have decreased to a very minimal level (Pan American Health Organization 1999).

Following the implementation of Law 100, Colombian's mental health system also became decentralized. Appropriations for mental health services are now passed through the departments. Each department has its own administrative health department, which transmits funding for psychiatric hospitals. Psychiatric hospitals are the main providers of mental health services for the general population and the indigent. They provide both inpatient and outpatient treatment. Health care providers (EPSs) also contract with psychiatric hospitals to serve their clientele.

Although this new system has definitely increased the use of primary care services, access to specialists has not similarly increased. In the case of mental health, no countrywide infrastructure is available that could facilitate increased access to psychiatric services. Resources for mental health services are scarce, and the development of a parallel national mental health plan seems to be badly needed.

ACCULTURATION AND MENTAL HEALTH SYMPTOMS

While investigating Colombians in New York, Correa (1992) found that acculturative stressors were better predictors of anxiety and depression than were general life stressors and also found that individuals who were more psychosocially competent used more active (problem-solving) coping strategies and experienced fewer symptoms of distress.

Patterns of migration and acculturation vary from one Colombian to another. Some live, work, and barely function, but avoid acculturation, refusing to learn English and living a Colombian lifestyle within the boundaries of their households. At the other extreme, some become very assimilated, marry Anglo-Saxons, and want little to do with their culture of origin. The majority, in the middle, become acculturated in various ways but struggle to preserve their original culture. Many travel frequently to Colombia to visit relatives, and the majority spend large amounts of money on telephone calls. Nostalgia is common, especially in males, whose desire to return tends to be greater than women's. The latter, especially those who suffered sexism in the old country, are very hesitant about going back to Colombia. However, the majority of Colombians frequently express nostalgia for the relatives and friends left behind. They accommodate by making new friends and by belonging to groups that can give them a little flavor of the past. Parties and family reunions are frequent. Immigrants also accommodate by joining civic organizations and by trying to bring other relatives to the United States, at whatever cost. Back-and-forth migration is not as prevalent as it is for other Hispanic groups.

Migration may cause grief, depression, nostalgia, distress, and, for some, trauma. Shame and guilt, two characteristics that tend to be common among Colombians, may contribute to complicating their psychological status, especially for those who have to perform work-related activities considered to be inferior in nature.

As the result of migration, some Colombian families tend to present marital conflicts, difficulties in communication with their teenage children, and symptoms of posttraumatic stress disorder. Alcoholism tends to be common in males; depression occurs frequently in women (Leon 1993). Colombians also show frequent symptoms of somatization, resulting from postmigration stress. Escobar (1987; Escobar et al. 1983) documented higher somatization indexes among Colombian patients with major depression compared to North American patients.

ATTITUDES TOWARD MENTAL HEALTH

Seeking the help of a psychiatrist is not the preferred line of action for Colombians going through emotional problems. Because the traditional belief system perceives psychiatrists as doctors who specialize in treating crazy people *(los loqueros)*, Colombians may exhibit a tendency to avoid mental health treatment. They tend to be more receptive to the words *counseling, orientation,* or *therapy.* This attitude prevents many from seeking treatment in a timely fashion. In this case, Colombians behave similarly to other Hispanic groups.

In general, the information available regarding use of mental health services indicates that the majority of Colombians with psychiatric disorders tend to consult with primary care providers or other specialists rather than with mental health professionals. Additionally, lack of medical insurance, the language barrier, and shame are factors that limit the use of mental health services. English-speaking, middle-class Colombians may show some preference for being treated by non-Colombian practitioners. Fearing a breach of confidentiality, Colombians tend to avoid participation in group treatment. The use of folk healers is still common in some areas of Colombia, as well as in the United States. The services of the different types of Colombians and other Hispanic healers that exist in most American major cities are used more frequently by immigrants with low income and low levels of education (Rojano 1993).

Mental Health Treatment of Colombian Patients

To work effectively with Colombian migrants, it is necessary to depart from traditional treatment modalities and to use more comprehensive and creative approaches. A four-dimensional evaluation is recommended:

- A traditional psychosocial assessment should be undertaken.
- Migration-acculturation: It is important to examine what stage of the migration-acculturation process the family is undergoing.
- Cultural and spiritual values: Research has demonstrated that immigrants who have a stronger native cultural identity acculturate more easily.
- Socioeconomic conditions: A full evaluation of socioeconomic conditions is mandatory. Special emphasis needs to be placed on assessing the family's available support system.

Interventions can take place at three levels: the individual, the familial, and the systemic-social. Individual interventions must be geared to helping clients deal with the losses related to migration and to overcoming any previous traumatic experience. Interventions must also reinforce self-esteem and help clients construct a system of beliefs that can help them acculturate, adapt, and cope.

Family interventions could help the couple renegotiate their traditional roles, establish new rules of the game, and learn new strategies and skills for effectively communicating with and disciplining their children. In general, family interventions try to help people develop the necessary flexibility to cope with new family roles and other demands of the new environment.

At the systemic level, a network intervention is almost mandatory. Clients or patients need to be helped not only to extend their social network but also to improve its quality, making it more functional for them. Strategies for increasing accessibility must be combined with interventions aimed at enhancing the use of the social support system. In the absence of families of origin, these networks are invaluable resources that have proved to enhance acculturation.

All of these strategies must be combined with other therapeutic approaches, depending on the availability of such services and the level of training and skill of the therapist. The following case example illustrates some of these ideas.

> Mr. C did not want to be in therapy. He still remembered the cold face of the social worker as she told him that he had to enter mandatory treatment or she would press charges against him. He kept thinking that if it were not for his wife's stubbornness, the family would already have moved back to Colombia. He had foreseen that bad things were going to happen to the family. As he expected, his 14-year-old daughter was "out of control." She no longer wanted to spend time with the family, she was hanging out with "bad company," and she was openly challenging her parents' authority.
>
> Mr. C did not think that things were working out well for him. Even though he had a well-paying job and was able to buy a house for his family, he felt basically discontented. He did admit that his financial condition was better than when he had migrated. Upon arriving in the United States, however, he had had to work odd jobs, and he had felt so humiliated by this that he was very careful to hide his employment from friends and family. Even though he was eventually able to obtain a better job, he did not feel that he was working at the level he thought he deserved.
>
> He was married to Mrs. C., whom he had met 4 years after migrating, while she was a tourist. They had had a brief courtship and married only 4 months after meeting. The honeymoon did not last long: they immediately begin to argue because he wanted to return to their country, whereas she wanted to stay in the United States. In time Mr. C begin to verbally abuse her, and he started drinking quite heavily; in the meantime she kept postponing their return home.
>
> At the time of treatment the couple had two children; a daughter, age 14, and a son, age 9. The couple was having a difficult time disciplining the children. The daughter perceived the family to be "boring," and she described her mother as always complaining and nagging and her father as "not caring" about anything. The parents attributed the problems they were having with their children as being the fault of the United States culture. For example, Mr. C was convinced that all the children needed was a good spanking; after all, this is how he and his wife had been disciplined when they were children. He remembered that when he had lived at home, all his father had to do was give him that special "look" and that was enough to make him behave.
>
> The distress between the parents and children was increasing, particularly with the daughter. They had decided to send her to Catholic school as a solution to their problems, but this did not help. Recently, Mr. C had learned that the daughter had lied about her whereabouts and had been in a car with friends. Mr. C decided to show her who was boss in the family. While he was scolding her, she raised her voice to him, and he felt that she had crossed the line. He took out his belt to use as a threat. When his own father had threat-

ened him with a belt, Mr. C was often able to avert a beating by asking for forgiveness. However, his daughter challenged him and in a defiant voice said, "If you dare to hit me I will call the police." And she did.

This case demonstrates a family who is experiencing difficulties at various levels. There is marital conflict and child-parent conflict. The family members as individuals also have various difficulties: the father is in emotional distress because he has made an incomplete transition to the host society, the mother has unspecified emotional problems, and the daughter is demonstrating oppositional behavior.

The approach used to treat this family was multidimensional. First, brief individual treatment was provided to the father with the goal of improving his self-esteem.

The assessment made of this family focused on their strengths. While making an inventory of their assets, it was found that they had many positive areas that they could draw on in times of crisis. First, they had a deep level of spirituality, were active in the church, and saw the priest as someone they could turn to for help. Because of this, they accepted the suggestion that they participate in one of the church's organized family retreats, where they would have the opportunity to talk to each other "from the soul." The retreat proved to be a good experience. Mr. C was able to apologize to his wife for his verbal mistreatment, and she forgave him. After the retreat they were more receptive to treatment and began couples therapy.

When the relationship between the couple began to improve, the daughter was brought into the sessions. It was obvious that the three had been feeling very alienated from each other, and they seemed to enjoy the opportunity to reengage in communication. For example, both parents were able to listen to the tips that their daughter gave them about how to handle a teenager in the United States. As part of the treatment, the daughter was referred to the school social worker, who helped her cope with school problems and who reinforced the family interventions.

The couple sessions continued to focus on both present problem solving and the resolution of past issues, such as how to enjoy life in the United States. Mrs. C decided to spend more time with her friends and to participate in some philanthropic activities, while Mr. C decided to become more active in a sports club. When on their own, they were able to negotiate reasonable plans about when to return to their country, they found they no longer needed therapy, and they decided to terminate treatment.

REFERENCES

Ardila R: Psicologia en Colombia: Contexto Social e Histórico, Primera Edición. Santa Fe de Bogota, Colombia, Tercer Mundo Editores, 1993

Correa M: Differences Among Colombian Immigrants in Coping and Distress: The Role of Personality and Stress. Doctoral dissertation, Long Island University, New York, 1992

Departamento Administrativo Nacional de Estadistica (DANE): Colombia Estadistica 1990, Vol 1. Santa Fe de Bogota, Colombia, DANE, Centro Administrativo Nacional (CAN), 1990

Departamento Administrativo Nacional de Estadistica (DANE): Información Estadística, 2001. Available at: http://www.dane.gov.co/Informacion_Estadistica/informacion_estadistica.html

Embassy of the Republic of Colombia to the United States: Colombia for Kids. Washington, DC, Embassy of Colombia, 2001. Available at: http://www.colombiaemb.org/English/Kids/kids.html

Escobar JI: Cross-cultural aspects of the somatization trait. Hospital and Community Psychiatry 38:174–180, 1987

Escobar JI, Gomez J, Tuason VB: Depressive phenomenology in North and South American patients. Am J Psychiatry 140:47–51, 1983

Europe World Book: Colombia statistical survey. London, England, Europe Publications, 2000

Forero J: Prosperous Colombians flee, many to U.S., to escape war. New York Times, April 10, 2001:A1

Gaviria C, et al: Constitucion Politica de Columbia. Santa Fe de Bogota, Colombia, Ediciones J Bernal, 1991

Grupo Temático de Desplazamiento: Datos sobre desplazamiento en Colombia, 2000. Available at: http://www.col.ops-oms.org/desplazados/cifras/default.htm

Gutierrez de Pineda V: Familia y Cultura en Colombia, Vol 2: Tipologias, Funciones y Dinamica de las Familias. Bogota, Instituto Colombiano de Cultura, 1975a

Gutierrez de Pineda V: Estructura, Funcion y Cambio de la Familia en Colombia. Bogota, Asociacion Colombiana de Facultades de Medicina, 1975b

Heaton TB, Chadwick BA, Jacobson CK: Statistical Handbook on Racial Groups in the United States. Westport, CT, Oryx Press, 2000

Inter-American Bank of Development: Gross domestic product per capita (table, in Keys to Latin American and the Caribbean 1999 (online book), 3rd Edition. Caracas, Venezuela, Sistema Económico Latinoamericano (SELA), May 1999. Available at: http://lanic.utexas.edu/project/sela/docs/claves99/keyslac/ameri.htm

Leon CA: The clinical profile of dysthymia in a group of Latin American women: worldwide therapeutic strategies in atypical depressive syndromes. European Psychiatry 8(5):252–255, 1993

Lopez C, Rojano R, et al: Algunas Caracteristicas Socioeconomicas y Culturales de las Familias del Area Urbana del Municipio de Medellin. Medellin, Colombia, Universidad de Antioquia, Facultad de Medicina, 1983

Pan American Health Organization (PAHO): Health Conditions in the Americas, Vols 1 and 2. Washington, DC, Scientific Publications of PAHO, 1994

Pan American Health Organization (PAHO): Colombia: Basic Country Health Profiles, Summaries, 1999 (online data). Washington, DC, Scientific Publications of PAHO, 1999. Available at: http://www.paho.org/English/SHA/prflcol.htm

Rojano R: El conflicto conyugal a traves del ciclo vital en Colombia. Revista Colombiana de Psiquiatria 14(4), 1985a

Rojano R: Problemas socioculturales de la familia y tres alternativas de la terapia de familia en Colombia. Revista Colombiana de Psiquiatria 14(1), 1985b

Rojano R: Migration and acculturation patterns of Colombian families in the United States. Paper presented at 32nd annual meeting of the Colombian Psychiatric Association, Medellin, Colombia, 1993

Seguridad Social en Colombia: Sistema Informativo de Seguridad Social en Colombia (Web site). Bogota, Colombia, 2001. Available at: http://www.ley100.com.co

Torres Y, Montoya I: Estudio Nacional de Salud Mental, 1997. Medellin, Colombia, Universidad Luis Amigo Press, 1997

U.S. Bureau of the Census: Statistical Abstract of the United States, 1993, 113th Edition. Washington, DC, U.S. Government Printing Office, 1993

U.S. Bureau of the Census: Statistical Abstract of the United States, 1998. Washington, DC, U.S. Government Printing Office, 1999

U.S. Bureau of the Census: World Population Profile: 1998 (Report WP/98). Washington, DC, U.S. Government Printing Office, 1999

U.S. Department of State: Background Notes: Colombia (online data). Washington, DC, U.S. Department of State, Bureau of Western Hemisphere Affairs, August 2000. Available at: http://www.state.gov/www/background_notes/colombia_0800_bgn.html

U.S. Library of Congress: Colombia: National Health Care System, in Library of Congress/Federal Research Division/Country Studies. Washington, DC, U.S. Library of Congress, 1998. Available at: http://lcweb2.loc.gov/frd/cs/cotoc.html#co0065

Velez L, McAllister A, et al: Measuring attitudes toward violence in Colombia. Journal of Social Psychology 137(4):533–534, 1997

World Book, Inc: Columbia, in World Book 2001, Vol 4. Chicago, IL, World Book Inc., 2001

CHAPTER 5

Cubans

Pedro Ruiz, M.D.

THE ISLAND OF CUBA is located in the Caribbean, approximately 90 miles south of Key West, Florida. It is approximately the size of the state of Tennessee. Currently, there are 10 million Cubans living on the island and 1 million living in the United States. In 1960 the racial composition of the 6.5 million Cubans on the island was 74% white, 11% black, 14% mulatto, and 1% Asian; 57% of the population lived in urban areas and 43% in rural. Additionally, there were 1.25 million workers unionized under a strong labor federation (Rumbaut 1990). The large majority of the Cuban population in Cuba and the Cuban-American population in the United States are Catholics (Rumbaut 1990).

HISTORICAL BACKGROUND

Christopher Columbus was the first European to arrive in Cuba, on October 27, 1492 (Rumbaut 1990). At the time of Columbus' arrival Cuba was inhabited by three Indian groups: the Guanahatabeyes, the Ciboneyes, and the Tainos. The Indian population of 60,000 was quickly eradicated by the disease that the Spaniards brought with them and by the imposition of slavery; thus a mere century after the discovery of Cuba only 5,000 Indians remained on the island. With the decline of this indigenous labor force, African slaves were brought into Cuba from the beginning of the eighteenth century through February 13, 1880 (Marquez Sterling and Marquez Sterling 1975).

Spain colonized Cuba from 1442 to 1899. The British also briefly occupied Cuba from 1762 to 1763. Cuba gained independence from Spain following a series of insurrections, three wars of independence, and the Spanish-American War of 1898–1899 (Thomas 1971). The United States occupied Cuba from 1899 to 1902 and later from 1906 to 1909. During this period the United States also tried to annex Cuba under the pretense of offering it the opportunity to prosper morally and materially (Thomas 1971). Presidents James Buchanan (1857–1861), Ulysses Grant (1869–1877), and William McKinley (1897–1901) also attempted to buy Cuba.

Cuba's democratic period, which started in 1902, has had several disruptions. The first of these was its occupation by the United States from 1906 to 1909. A right-wing dictatorship from 1929 to 1933 was followed by a series of interim governments. Later the government was again taken over by a right-wing dictatorship, from 1952 to 1959. The current left-wing dictatorship has been in place since 1959 (Thomas 1971). In many ways, the history of Cuba during the past 150 years explains the ambivalent feelings Cubans have toward the United States, the weakness of the Cuban political system throughout the years, and the inability of Cuba to achieve full democracy.

CUBAN MIGRATION TO THE UNITED STATES

Cuban Americans currently represent the third largest Hispanic group in the United States, with a population of about 1,053,197 million people, or 4.8% of the total United States population. Cuban Americans have settled in all major urban areas throughout the United States, but particularly in the states of Florida, New Jersey, and New York.

The first major wave of Cuban migration occurred during the second half of the nineteenth century, when approximately 100,000 Cubans left the island for political reasons and came to the United States (Gonzalez 1995). These Cubans settled primarily in New York City and in Tampa, Key West, and other Florida cities, where they established the tobacco industry (Diaz 1981). By the beginning of 1959, when Castro took control of Cuba, there were already 200,000 Cuban Americans living in the United States.

The early Cuban migrants fell into three categories. The first was made up of those who were unskilled workers and came chiefly from rural Cuba. Second was the professional group, mainly health care providers, who came to this country to obtain specialized medical training or financial security. Finally, there were the workers from the tobacco industry (Ruiz 1982).

Since Castro took control of the Cuban government in 1959, several waves of Cuban migration to the United States have taken place:

- The first occurred from 1959 to 1965, when about 183,400 Cubans arrived in this country (Jorge and Moncarz 1980). This group was primarily composed of white, educated upper-class or middle-class persons. These migrants usually had business and financial resources and a set of values and beliefs shared with the majority United States culture. Upon arriving in the United States, these Cubans received massive financial and educational support from the United States government (Bernal and Estrada 1985; Cortes 1980; Prohias and Casal 1980).
- The second took place during the period 1965–1973, when approximately 264,300 Cubans entered the United States (Jorge and Moncarz 1980). This group was primarily composed of white adult women from middle-class, lower middle-class, or working-class Cuba.
- The third, known as the Mariel boat lift, took place in 1980, when about 125,000 Cubans migrated. They were primarily a working-class population. However, a small group of these migrants included "antisocial" and mentally ill individuals purposely sent to the United States by the Cuban government (Bernal 1982).
- The last took place in 1995, when about 25,000 Cubans left the island via small boats, rafts, and floats.

CUBANS IN THE UNITED STATES

The settlement of Cuban Americans in the United States has resulted in the evolution of five socioeconomic groups. The Cuban aristocracy and bourgeoisie, who had ties to United States capital and business before Castro took over Cuba, represent about 25,000 families, or 1% of the Cuban workforce in the United States. The upper-middle-class sector, composed of professionals and small-business owners, represent about 18% of this workforce. Salaried professionals, technicians, and administrators and managers make up the middle class, which is 21% of this workforce. The majority of Cuban Americans (60%) are in the working class, composed of salaried workers in the production of materials, the service sector, and the office sector. Finally, there is a very small antisocial sector, many of whom have close connections to organized crime in this country (Valdez-Paz and Hernandez 1984). Unlike the majority of Hispanic American groups who have settled in the United States, Cuban Americans tend to be very conservative and usually vote for the Republican Party (Bernal and Gutierrez 1988).

Socioeconomically, Cubans in the United States have done well, with perhaps the exception of those who entered via the 1980 Mariel boat lift (Portes 1987; Portes et al. 1985). This stable economic status has allowed Cubans to fare better than other Hispanic groups in the United States, as indicated in Table 5–1 (U.S. Bureau of the Census 1991).

Table 5–1. Socioeconomic and educational data on three Hispanic groups in the United States

	Cuban Americans (%)	Mexican Americans (%)	Puerto Ricans (%)	Total U.S. population (%)
Family below poverty level	15.2	28.4	33	12.8
Income less than $10,000/year	12.2	18.6	28	9.9
Income more than $50,000/year	23.5	12.6	15.4	29
Female head of household	18.9	19.5	38.9	16.5
High school diploma	63.5	44.1	55.5	77.6
College degree	20.2	5.4	9.7	21.3

Source. U.S. Bureau of the Census 1991.

ALCOHOL AND SUBSTANCE USE

Cuban Americans' socioeconomic conditions have permitted them to do well with respect to access to health and mental health services (Ruiz 1994; Ruiz et al. 1995). It has been found that the incidence of psychiatric illness among Cuban Americans does not differ from its incidence among other Hispanic-American subgroups, with the exception of substance abuse and alcoholism.

Ruiz and Langrod (1982) found differences in the use of alcohol, marijuana, and cocaine among Cuban Americans, Mexican Americans, and Puerto Ricans. They found that 59.8% of Cuban Americans abstain from alcohol consumption, compared with 50.3% of Mexican Americans and 59.6% of Puerto Ricans. Cuban Americans also drink at a lower rate compared with the other two groups. The rate of cocaine use is much lower among Cuban Americans (9.2%) than among Mexican Americans (11.1%) or Puerto Ricans (21.5%). Similarly, the rate of marijuana use is lower among Cuban Americans (20.1%) than among Mexican Americans (41.6%) or Puerto Ricans (42.7%). It has been stated that among Cuban Americans, acculturation patterns, along the lines of integration, could have a protective role against drug or alcohol use (Ruiz 1994).

Sokol-Katz and Ulbrich (1992) studied the alcohol consumption and drug use patterns of Cuban American, Mexican American, and Puerto Rican adolescents. They found that the rate of alcohol consumption was higher among Cuban Americans (16.1%) than among Mexican Americans (14.7%) or

Puerto Ricans (11.7%). Cuban American youth had a lower rate of drug use (15%) than either Mexican Americans (29.7%) or Puerto Ricans (28.4%). It was also found that Cuban American adolescents who preferred to speak English had the highest rates of alcohol consumption and drug use. The family structure had no effect on alcohol or drug use among Cuban American adolescents, whereas Mexican American and Puerto Rican adolescents living in female-headed households had a higher risk.

PSYCHIATRIC CLINICAL CONSIDERATIONS

Stigma plays a major role in the treatment of mental illness in Cuba and among Cuban Americans; culturally, the connotation of being "crazy" is not well accepted (Bernal 1985). In Cuba, psychiatry and mental illness are primarily associated with the Mazorra, a hospital where both the environment and the care were abysmal until the early 1960s (Camayd-Freixas and Uriarte 1980). As a result, many Cubans and Cuban Americans prefer to seek psychiatric care from family doctors (Rogg and Coney 1980). Fortunately, there has been an improvement in the mental health system in Cuba, and much emphasis is now given to community-based treatment (Kates 1987). The exception to this rule is the physical and mental health treatment rendered to persons infected with HIV-1 in Cuba. The Cuban government has implemented a mass testing campaign on the island, and persons found to be infected with the HIV-1 virus or to have AIDs are placed under mandatory quarantine (Pérez-Stable 1991).

As with other Hispanic groups, it is important to consider that Cuban Americans often do not distinguish between illness and disease. *Disease* is generally perceived as a malfunction of the biological-physiological process, whereas *illness* encompasses personal, interpersonal, and environmental reactions and functions (Ruiz 1994). Perhaps this is one of the reasons why many Cuban Americans seek treatment for their mental illness among spiritual healers. Generally, folk and spiritual healers emphasize illness and thus give their patients a more acceptable explanation of psychiatric problems and conditions. Folk-healing traditions combining African religious beliefs with Catholicism remain prominent in certain sectors of the Cuban American population as well as in Cuba. These unorthodox religious beliefs are manifested in the practice of *Santeria,* spiritism, and *brujeria* (Bernal and Gutierrez 1988; Ruiz 1982, 1994). *Santeria* is a folk religion in which Yoruba deities originally from Africa are identified with Catholic saints. Spiritism involves belief in the existence of spirits and their communication with the visible world. *Brujeria* is synonymous with witchcraft and regards illnesses as being caused by natural or supernatural forces.

Several clinical issues should be considered when psychiatrically assessing and treating Cuban American patients:

- Be aware of Cuban Americans' culture and historical background.
- Recognize the role of acculturation among Cuban Americans.
- Evaluate the socioeconomic and class status of Cuban American patients and how status affects their health care and mental health care.
- Be aware of the high rate of alcoholism among Cuban American adolescents.
- Evaluate the role of religion in the life of Cuban American patients and how religion affects their health care and mental health care.
- Incorporate the nuclear and extended family network into mental health treatment.
- Use psychosocial education to combat the stigma of mental illness and treatment.
- Be aware of the tendency to somatize among Cuban American patients.
- Explore Cuban Americans' understanding of the etiology of their mental illness and act accordingly.

The following case example points up some of the areas discussed here.

The patient was a self-referred middle-aged Cuban American black male sociologist whose presenting problem was "impotence." He had heard about me from a friend of his, whom I had treated in the past.

The patient asked for psychiatric consultation and treatment because he had been experiencing progressive impotence for 2–3 months. At the onset of the illness he was able to sustain partial erections and to have intercourse, but during the last month he had been unable to have an erection.

He denied any previous history of psychiatric illness or treatment. He also did not report a history of serious medical or surgical illnesses. As a child, he had had the usual childhood illnesses, and he denied a history of traumas, injuries, or allergic reactions. He did acknowledge that he had not had a physical checkup in 3–4 years and that during the preceding 3 months he had been having frequency of urination. He denied any history of substance use but acknowledged that he drank socially. He had never been drunk.

The patient was raised in Cuba and lived in a Catholic home with his parents and four siblings. He described a happy childhood and denied a history of sexual or physical abuse or school problems. He started masturbating at age 12 and began dating at age 15. He married at age 26, after he had finished his university studies in Cuba, and he reported that he had had a happy marriage until he started experiencing impotence. He had and his wife had no children.

At the time of seeking treatment, the patient had been living in the United States for 20 years. He was working for the government as a sociologist, and his wife was a teacher's aide in the public school system. He had no history of being arrested or ever being involved with the criminal justice system. He also had no history of military service.

The patient did not have information about the status of his family because they were still in Cuba; however, he did know that his father had died of a heart attack several years ago. He did not know of any family history of psychiatric illness.

During a review of symptoms, the patient reported an increase in appetite for 2–3 months and a weight gain of 20 pounds during that period. He also reported waking up frequently during the night for about 1 month. As previously mentioned, he also reported frequency of urination.

I referred the patient to a family physician for a complete physical examination and laboratory workup. I requested attention to the possible existence of diabetes mellitus. The diagnostic test was requested by the family practitioner and showed a mild increase in blood glucose level. All other tests were normal, including an electrocardiogram and chest X rays.

In the mental status examination, the patient appeared moderately overweight, anxious, and concerned about his sexual problems. His mood was somewhat depressed and his affect normal. He was goal directed in his communication pattern and showed a normal speech rate. His thought content and perception were normal except for his excessive worries about sexual dysfunction. He denied suicidal or homicidal ideation, obsessions, compulsions, phobias, or panic attacks. The Mini-Mental State Exam (Folstein et al. 1975) showed his cognition to be intact; he was oriented, his remote and recent memory were intact, and his judgment was not impaired. He also demonstrated good insight in that he accepted the finding that his problem must be treated both medically and psychiatrically.

His main complaint was feeling somewhat depressed and anxious. He worried about his loss of "masculinity" due to his the impotence and about what his wife's potential reactions would be if he were not cured soon. He saw his tension and anxiety as contributing to his sleep difficulties and overeating.

After a through psychiatric assessment and the completion of the medical workup, I formulated the following DSM-IV diagnoses:

Axis I: Adjustment disorder with mixed anxiety and depressed mood
Axis II: None
Axis III: Diabetes mellitus, mild
Axis IV: Psychosocial stressors: problems related to his sexual functioning
Axis V: GAF = −65 (at time of the assessment)

The case formulation is shown in the following paragraphs.

Traditional formulation. The recent loss of sexual power (erection) acted as a strong stressor to which the patient had to adapt. Subsequently, his mood and anxiety became very prominent because of the psychological traumatic event suffered. The diabetes mellitus also played a major factor in the patient's sexual problems.

Cultural formulation. Identity of the individual: the patient was born and raised in Cuba. He migrated to the United States when he was in his early thirties. He lived in a heavily populated Hispanic neighborhood and had retained his native culture and heritage.

Cultural explanation of the individual illness. Culturally, the loss of erection and thus impotence in a Cuban American black male acted as a major trauma. The perception of being *macho* (masculine) is threatened when erection problems develop. This situation can easily lead to adjustment problems, major depression, and even suicide if not appropriately and quickly treated.

Cultural factors related to psychosocial environment and levels of functioning. The Hispanic values associated with masculinity *(machismo),* with its inherent cultural connotations, played a significant role in the patient's reactions and illness. Hopefully, his extended network system permitted him to seek health services promptly.

Cultural elements of the relationship between the individual and the clinician. The fact that I am Hispanic and Cuban American myself permitted me to understand quickly the culturally rooted stressors that the patient was suffering. This understanding helped to cement a good doctor-patient relationship, on which the outcome of treatment was dependent.

Overall cultural assessment for diagnoses and care. The cultural milieu in which the patient and the therapist (myself) were raised allowed an excellent rapport and quick understanding to develop. This in turn permitted a prompt medical-psychiatric intervention, thus avoiding a severe progression of the medical illness (diabetes mellitus) and the psychiatric condition (depression, with possibility of suicide). The following cultural factors played a significant role in this case: *machismo,* an extended network system, the bilinguality and biculturality of the therapist, and finally the patient's prompt seeking of physical health and mental health services.

The clinical intervention is described below:

> I started out by seeing the patient twice a week for 1 month and once a week thereafter until I began to gradually discontinue treatment 3 months later. I saw him every 2 weeks for 1 month, then once a month for 2 months. From the time of evaluation, I saw him for a total of 6 months.
>
> Initially, I prescribed 25 mg of Atarax (hydroxyzine hydrochloride) at bedtime. In therapy I focused on building the doctor-patient relationship

and on gaining his trust. I acknowledged his problems and demonstrated an understanding of his fear about the potential of permanently losing his masculinity (erection) and possibly his wife. At the same time I stressed that his marriage had lasted for 30 years and that his wife had always been on his side. I also emphasized that she had even left her family behind in Cuba to accompany him to the United States. In therapy I also reinforced the fact that the diabetes mellitus was playing a major role in his sexual dysfunction. This helped to alleviate his guilt feelings and permitted him to focus on a material cause for his sexual dysfunction, rather than on a more abstract psychological one.

His family practitioner placed him on hypoglycemic medications and a 1,200-calorie diet. I also encouraged him to join an athletic club for the purpose of losing weight, building a strong body and muscles, and raising his spirits. After 2 months I discontinued the Atarax, since he was sleeping well and his anxiety had greatly diminished. After 3 months he had lost about 20 pounds and regained his erection capability, and all the stress disappeared.

I based my psychological interventions on cognitive and supportive psychotherapy. After 4 months, I started working on termination and separation issues, and treatment was terminated at 6 months. Upon the patient's discharge, I asked the family practitioner to give me a call if he saw a reemergence of the anxiety or depressive symptoms. I also told the client to call me if any of the problems he had been having recurred.

Without question, my cultural understanding of this Cuban American patient permitted me to successfully treat him with minimal intervention, in a brief, cost-effective manner. It also prevented the development of a more severe depression, even potentially suicide. Moreover, it helped me in getting quick access to physical health services and the treatment of his diabetes mellitus, again in a biculturally sensitive milieu.

REFERENCES

Bernal G: Cuban families (Chapter 9), in Ethnicity and Family Therapy. Edited by McGoldrick M, Pearce JK, Giordano J. New York, Guilford, 1982

Bernal G: A History of Psychology in Cuba. Journal of Community Psychology 13:222–234, 1985

Bernal G, Estrada A: Cuban Refugee and Minority Experiences: A Book Review. Hispanic Journal of Behavioral Sciences 7:105–128, 1985

Bernal G, Gutierrez M: Cubans, in Clinical Guidelines in Cross-Cultural Mental Health. Edited by Comas-Diaz L, Griffith EEH. New York, Wiley, 1988, pp 233–261

Camayd-Freixas Y, Uriarte M: The Organization of Mental Health Services in Cuba. Hispanic Journal of Behavioral Sciences 2:337–354, 1980

Cortes CE (ed): The Cuban Experience in the United States. New York, Arno, 1980

Diaz GM: The changing Cuban community, in Hispanics and Grantmakers: A Special Report of Foundation News. Washington, DC, Council on Foundations, 1981, pp 18–23

Folstein MF, Folstein SE, McHugh PR: "Mini-Mental State": a practical method for grading the cognitive state of patients for the clinician. J Psychiatr Res 12:189–198, 1975

Gonzalez GM: Cuban-Americans, in Experiencing and Counseling Multicultural and Diverse Populations, 3rd Edition. Edited by Vace NA, DeVaney SB, Wittmer J. Bristol, PA, Taylor & Francis, 1995, pp 293–316

Jorge A, Moncarz R: Cubans in south Florida: a social science approach. Metas 1:37–87, 1980

Kates N: Mental Health Services in Cuba. Hospital and Community Psychiatry 38:755–758, 1987

Marquez Sterling C, Marquez Sterling M: Historia de La Isla de Cuba. New York, Regents Publishing, 1975

Pérez-Stable E: Cuba's response to the HIV epidemic. Am J Public Health 81:563–567, 1991

Portes A: The social origins of the Cuban enclave economy of Miami. Sociological Perspectives 30(4):340–372, 1987

Portes A, Clark JM, Manning RD: After Mariel: a survey of the resettlement experiences of 1980 Cuban refugees in Miami. Cuban Studies/Estudios Cubanos 15(2):37–59, 1985

Prohias RJ, Casal L (eds): The Cuban Minority in the United States. New York, Arno, 1980

Rogg EM, Coney RS: Adaptation and Adjustment of Cubans: West New York, New Jersey (Monograph, No 5). Bronx, New York, Hispanic Research Center, Fordham University, 1980

Ruiz P: Cuban-Americans, in Cross-Cultural Psychiatry. Edited by Gaw A. Boston, MA, John Wright-PSG, 1982, pp 75–86

Ruiz P: Cuban Americans: migration, acculturation, and mental health, in Theoretical and Conceptual Issues in Hispanic Mental Health. Edited by Malgady RG, Rodriguez O. Malabar, FL, Krieger Publishing, 1994, pp 70–89

Ruiz P, Langrod J: Cultural issues in the mental health of Hispanics in the United States. American Journal of Social Psychiatry 2:35–38, 1982

Ruiz P, Venegas-Samuels K, Alarcón RD: the economics of pain: mental health care costs among minorities. Psychiatr Clin North Am 18:649–670, 1995

Rumbaut RD: Cuba's fate: a lesson for modern world? Texas Catholic Herald, June 22, 1990, p 16

Sokol-Katz JS, Ulbrich PT: Family structure and adolescent risk-taking behavior: a comparison of Mexican, Cuban, and Puerto Rican Americans. Int J Addict 23:1197–1209, 1992

Thomas H: Cuba: The pursuit of freedom. New York, Harper & Row, 1971

U.S. Bureau of the Census: Current Population Report, Series P-20, No 499. Washington, DC, U.S. Department of Commerce, Bureau of the Census, 1991

Valdez-Paz J, Hernandez R: La estructura social de la comunidad Cubana en Estados Unidos, in Cubans in the United States. Edited by Uriarte-Gaston M, Cañas-Martinez J. Boston, MA, Center for the Study of the Cuban Community, 1984

CHAPTER 6

Dominicans

Carmen Inoa Vazquez, Ph.D., A.B.P.P.

THE DOMINICAN REPUBLIC HAS been known by various names during the various periods of its history. It was called Quisqueya by the Indians, Española or Little Spain by the Spaniards (later anglicized to La Hispaniola), and Santo Domingo (Saint Domingue) by the Haitians (Wiarda 1969).

A part of the West Indies, the Dominican Republic shares the island of La Hispaniola with Haiti. It occupies two-thirds of the island. The Dominican Republic is located southeast of Cuba and west of Puerto Rico. It extends north to the Atlantic Ocean and south to the Caribbean Sea.

The population of the Dominican Republic is approximately 7,515,892, and it continues to grow at a rapid pace. The age structure of the population has been changing since the 1970s. There has been a decline in infants and young people, with an increase in middle-aged persons. In 1993, the age distribution was 36% ages 9–14, 60% ages 15–64, and only 4% over age 65 (Plan Nacional de Salud Mental 1995).

The economy and demographics of the Dominican Republic have undergone great transformation since the mid-1980s. Although 1984–1985 was characterized as economically stable, the following 5 years were marked by a disequilibrium that affected the public sector, creating a 42% decline in the minimum wage and a 27% rise in unemployment. The contradictions in the economy are many. The people of the Dominican Republic are poor, but the land itself is rich in bauxite, nickel, and gold. Although industry employs a steadily growing number of people, approximately four out of five Dominicans derive their living from agriculture; sugar cane, cacao, and coffee are the main export crops. The valleys of Cibao and the Vega Real are heavily populated and the country's primary source of agricultural wealth. However, the Dominican Republic has quite rapidly changed from a country with a predominantly rural population to one in which urban and rural populations are almost evenly divided: currently, the population distribution is 52% rural and 48% urban.

The most densely populated urban area is the capital or National District, with a population of 819/square mile. The *campesinos* (peasants) who have been expelled from rural areas have been forced to move to the cities, where they have become a marginalized people.

The population is composed of three major ethnic groups: Indians (the indigenous people), Europeans, and Africans. However, Dominicans for the most part are racially mixed. During the early part of the Spanish rule, miscegenation between Europeans and Indians and between Africans and Indians was widespread. The original indigenous population of Hispaniola was eradicated, and there are now few remnants of the original Caribitaino and Arawak races and cultures. African slaves replaced the indigenous Indians in the culture, and eventually the African population outnumbered the Spanish by approximately 2:1. Dominicans, however, speak Spanish and are anthropologically depicted as culturally Hispanic.

DOMINICAN CULTURE AND RELIGION

Catholicism is the official religion of the Dominican Republic; Protestants did not arrive on the island until the 1820s. A formal division between church and state exists, but in certain aspects this division becomes diffuse. For example, there is no need to marry in a civil court if the marriage is conducted in the Catholic Church. It is important to note that present popular religious beliefs, or *religiosidad popular Dominicana,* a mixture of mystical African beliefs and values with Catholicism, play a central role among Dominicans (Tejada Ortiz et al. 1993).

Similar to any other group, there is no specific Dominican "type" that could describe the entire Dominican population. However, Dominicans share certain basic concepts, including *machismo, marianismo, personalismo, familism,* and *respeto.* Dominicans value highly the dignity of the individual and the respect of others. *Familism* is based on the centrality of the family for Dominicans. *Machismo* and *marianismo* may be displayed in positive and negative forms. *Marianismo* is a specifically prescribed code of behaviors that apply to women. It includes norms of passivity, deference, and courtesy. These traditional cultural expectations require that women be stoic and capable of withstanding a great deal of suffering. At times, *marianismo* imposes the acceptance of very difficult behaviors from relatives and/or friends. *Machismo* in its negative form is all about rigid stereotypes that require specific behaviors that can limit tenderness and an array of other behaviors for men. These stereotypes define the place of a woman, including the way men should be served. *Machismo* can condone oppression of women, selfishness, and womanizing. But like *marianismo, machismo* has a positive side that includes responsibility, protection, and discipline. *Respeto* is a very central concept in the Latino culture that tells us how to interact with others and how others should interact with us (Gil and Vazquez 1996).

History and Migration

Christopher Columbus first colonized the Dominican Republic for Spain in 1492. It is believed that his remains are buried in the Faro a Colon (Columbus Lighthouse). Early in the colonial period, Santo Domingo was called the Cradle of America because it was used as the starting point for the exploration and conquests of other islands. Spain's initial interest in the island arose because of the discovery of gold there. During the early Spanish rule, schools and convents were built in Santo Domingo. Literature, theater, architecture, and the arts flourished, but once the gold supplies were exhausted, the Spaniards began to neglect the island. In 1795, the French who controlled the eastern part of the island, Saint Domingue, took possession of the entire island. Haiti, in turn, became independent from France in 1804 and in 1822 took over the eastern part of the island. Haitian domination lasted for 22 years, until 1844, when the part of the island known today as the Dominican Republic became an independent nation. Political upheaval and economic instability ensued for several years, eventually leading to partial control of the country by the United States, with an occupation by the U.S. Marines from 1916 to 1924. Six years after the marines left the Dominican Republic, Rafael Trujillo became president, staying in power as a dictator for 31 years (Bosch 1984; Moya Pons 1984; Urena 1966).

The Dominican Republic has a large immigrant population from Haiti. Statistics do not account for the total numbers, because they do not reflect illegal entry; however, it is estimated that there are 500,000–1,000,000 Haitians currently living in the country. The internal migration in the Dominican Republic from rural to urban zones is approximately 100,000/year; most of these people go to the capital (Plan Nacional de Salud Mental 1995). The statistics of international immigration are also imprecise, because a part of this immigration is illegal as well. According to some estimates, at least 1 million Dominicans have immigrated to the United States since the 1950s (Pellerano & Herrera 2001).

Despite the large number of Dominicans now living in the United States, there is little known about their characteristics and the composition of the Dominican diaspora. However, it is known that the Dominican immigrant flow is not one-directional (Cosgrove 1992). It is customary for Dominicans to move between the United States and their homeland, and it is estimated that approximately 25% of Dominican immigrants return to their homeland and that one-third of this group leaves their country again.

Dominicans in the United States have formed enclaves, particularly in the New York–New Jersey region (Bray 1987). North Manhattan has the largest concentration of Dominicans in New York City, a large number of them undocumented workers. Dominicans immigrate to the United States primarily for economic reasons, even though they often undergo a lowering of their occupational status and have difficulties adapting to their new host culture.

Adaptation to life in the United States has not been easy for Dominicans. They face problems of unemployment, underemployment, poor housing, lack of knowledge of English, and lack of adequate health services. This difficulty in adjustment is most predominant among professional male immigrants, because they often can only obtain nonskilled employment, usually in New York's garment district. Dominican males have one of the highest unemployment rates in New York City (Rodriguez et al. 1995). Migration has disrupted family units, separating spouses from each other and parents from children. The result has been high divorce rates, as well as high levels of stress and depression (Cosgrove 1992).

HEALTH SYSTEM

The Dominican Republic does not have a unified system of health services. Services are provided in a structure that includes the public and private sectors; also playing a part is the traditional medicine *curanderismo,* a system of self-medication in which individuals use common knowledge to determine what type of herbs or *tizanas* (tea brews) will cure a specific ailment or stressful situation.

As a result of Dominican participation in the 1990 Conference of Caracas, and an agreement between the Secretaria de Estado de Salud Publica y Asistencia Social (State Office of Public Health and Public Assistance), the Centro Colaborador de la Organizacion Mundial de la Salud de Venezia Giulia Italia—Instituto Franco Rotelli (Collaborating Center of the World

Health Organization of Venezia Giulia—Italy-Franco Institute), and the Organizacion Panamericana de la Salud (Pan-American Health Organization), efforts have been made to provide alternative treatment centers geared toward prevention and rehabilitation. Toward this end, the Ministry of Health SESPAS also offers psychiatric services in different general hospitals in the area of Santo Domingo, where ambulatory services are provided in mental health. Similarly, a number of units that provide community mental health services have been added to provide services in poor areas in various provinces throughout the nation. Services now include rehabilitation and the integration of families into the treatment of those patients who require electroconvulsive therapy (Plan Nacional de Salud Mental 1995).

The public (state) health sector has three components:

1. the State Office of Public Health and Public Assistance (La Secretaria de Estado de Salud Publica y Asistencia Social, or SESPAS), the government body responsible for providing services to the entire Dominican population

2. the Dominican Institute of Social Service (El Instituto Dominicano de Seguros Sociales, or IDSS), which is responsible for serving the health needs of workers that earn less than a certain amount, which in 1995 was $2,019 monthly

3. the Institute for Social Services of the Armed Forces and National Police (Instituto de Seguridad Social de las Fuerzas Armadas y la Policia Nacional, or SSFAPOL), which is responsible for providing services for those in the armed forces and the national police and their families

These institutions include health regions that provide services to rural clinics, local hospitals, and regional and national hospitals.

The SESPAS provides outpatient psychiatric services in various general hospitals located in urban areas. The Hospital Padre Billini is the primary psychiatric hospital in the entire nation. The staff is composed of approximately 25 psychiatrists, 3 psychologists, and 134 nurses. The hospital maintains minimal contact with communities and other medical facilities. The fact that there is only one psychiatric hospital to serve the entire nation clearly illustrates the need to place a higher priority on mental health services (Plan Nacional de Salud Mental 1995).

TRAINING OF MENTAL HEALTH PROVIDERS

The training of Dominican mental health providers takes place in either state-funded or private centers of learning. In 2001, nine major universities in the

Dominican Republic offered formal training in health services (Consejo Nacional de Educación Superior [CONES] 2001). The major center for training mental health providers is the Universidad Autonoma de Santo Domingo, which trains both psychiatrists and psychologists. However, other universities, such as the Universidad Catolica Madre y Maestra (UCAMAIMA) and the Universidad Iberoamericana, also provide training for mental health professionals. Currently, there is no formal training for social workers or for psychiatric nurses in the Dominican Republic. The main site offering residency training for psychiatrists is the State Psychiatric Hospital Padre Billini. This hospital has a chronic population, offering few preventive treatments and most of the treatment is of an episodic nature. Another major site also offering residency training in psychiatry is the State Hospital Salvador Gautier.

The Dominican Republic participated in the 1988–1990 Conference of Caracas, where mental health providers formulated goals and objectives to prioritize mental health training and to improve the coordination between universities that specialize in mental health training.

GENERAL BELIEFS ABOUT MENTAL ILLNESS

There is diversity among Dominicans, defined by region, socioeconomic status, and social class. It is therefore difficult to come up with a description of the culture that encompasses all Dominicans. However, certain characteristics of some groups of Dominicans cannot be ignored when providing mental health services.

As previously mentioned, popular religious practices play a central role in Dominican life. *Religiosidad popular Dominicana* includes a mixture of mystical African values and Catholicism, including spiritism such as Dominican voodoo, *curanderismo,* and the messianic movement. Manifestations of this mixture of religious beliefs are seen in such practices such as *el santiguo* (blessings by the sign of the cross), *curaciones* (healings of all illnesses, including mental illness), and other magical rituals (Zaglul 1993) involved in taking a mental patient to a *cuandera* (healer). The *cuandera* may offer special prayers; recommend baths with herbs, perfume, and/or flowers to purify the person; and in some special cases provide some type of exorcism. Another magical ritual is the *toque de manos,* a practice that was used by the kings of England and France. The *toque de manos* may include also the *santiguo* (blessing) and consist of rubbing the hands until they get hot and then placing them on the part of the body affected. Currently used in the Christian religions, including catholicism, *sanidad divina* (divine healing) is a practice based on healing achieved through prayers. These prayers may come from the individual who is seeking to be cured, or they may be offered in groups formed by members of a particular religious community or by family members or friends.

In certain parts of the country, when someone dies, all receptacles that contain water must be emptied immediately lest the soul bathe in any of the receptacles intended for drinking water. Similarly, if, on the way to the cemetery, the coffin bearers stop in front of a house where there is an ill person, the person must get up immediately from the bed to avoid death. To sleep with the feet facing the street attracts death; wearing black to a wedding causes bad luck. It is common for legislators and politicians to consult *brujos* (witches and warlords) for advice and to wear *resguardos* (amulets). Even in the homes of wealthier Dominicans it is not unusual to find a little corner of the house adorned with flowers and lit candles (Tejada Ortiz et al. 1993). *Resguardos* guard against evil and illness. Illnesses such as colds or evil spirits can be warded off by *azabaches,* black onyx amulets; crosses made out of anil or indigo; and *resguardos* made out of camphor salts. *Agua de Florida,* an eau de cologne splashed or sprayed on to cool the body and refresh the senses, is thought to disperse negative influences and is used to cure headaches, hives, and skin rashes. The *ensalmo* (blessing) is used to cure swollen glands, *hernia empachos* (stomach problems), and many other ailments.

RECOMMENDATIONS FOR CLINICIANS

It is important to recognize that as a result of the constant contact that Dominicans in the United States retain with the Dominican Republic, their acculturation may differ from that of other Hispanics in the United States. The remigration process puts Dominicans in double jeopardy, because they feel marginalized and unintegrated in both the United States and the Dominican Republic. Remigration may make the process of acculturation not only difficult but at times improbable, as exemplified by the significant levels of maladjustment (Cosgrove 1992). Unemployment and the lowering of occupational status, particularly in professional men, can cause significant stresses among family members, aggravating the possibility of domestic violence, alcoholism, and negative effects on both marital relationships and parent-child relationships.

In assessment of Dominicans in psychiatric settings, it is important for clinicians to consider the following points:

- Dominicans adhere to traditional Hispanic cultural values regarding family, gender role expectations, *machismo,* and *marianismo.*
- Religion is important to most Dominicans and salient in their therapy.

- Families migrate at different times, creating different levels of acculturation. This discrepancy in acculturation may cause friction between adolescents and their parents.
- Young children and adolescents may experience difficulty acculturating at school and with friends, as well as integrating their two cultures.
- Fear of deportation often results in women denying being victims of domestic violence.
- Clinicians working with Dominicans should not try to impose one culture over another; instead, they need to help clients integrate both cultures in a functional manner.

The following case example illustrates how environment, culture, and health care beliefs can interface. Many Dominicans share values and a belief system that must be understood in the context of the process of acculturation to the host culture. Many of these values and beliefs can be specific to the immigration experience, while others can be part of the overall Latino experience in the United States. Similar to other immigrants, Dominicans bring with them a specific worldview.

> Mr. D is a 38-year-old Dominican male working as a caseworker in a mental health clinic in the Bronx. He completed medical school in the Dominican Republic, but he could not find a residency in the United States despite knowing English well. His wife is a 35-year-old Dominican working at the United Nations as an administrative assistant.
>
> Mr. D came to therapy at Mrs. D's insistence. She reported that he had distanced himself from her, that he seemed sad and irritable, and that he did not have the same energy level he had possessed in the Dominican Republic. She further reported that the couple no longer shared common pleasures. Mr. D no longer liked to entertain at home, which made her feel isolated. Furthermore, she was unhappy because she did not feel that Mr. D understood how difficult it was for her to work outside the home, manage the household, and take care of the children without outside assistance.
>
> Mr. D complained that Mrs. D was argumentative and had become "too Americanized." He reported that she insisted on going to the gym and out with her friends, instead of taking care of the children. And to make matters worse, she expected Mr. D to care for the children in her absence. He complained that Mrs. D did not understand how hard he had to work outside the home.

What we see in the above example is a brief illustration of some of the stresses that immigration and acculturation can create in a marital relationship. Mrs. D is experiencing a crisis in both her marriage and her adaptation to her new culture. She feels incompetent, guilty, sad, and overwhelmed.

Mr. D, who has suffered the loss of occupational status as a result of immigration, also feels sad, as well as incompetent because he is unable to provide for his family as he did in the Dominican Republic. He feels threatened by the changes in Mrs. D and the new demands she makes on him. His sense of *machismo* (masculinity) is affected because his wife now works outside the home. The idea of helping with the household and the children is culturally dissonant to him.

The therapist helped Mr. D understand that the process of acculturation was not easy for himself, his wife, or any other person in their situation. Mr. D was helped to adapt to his new role and to understand the painful reality of being unable to practice his profession or to take care of his family in a culturally consonant manner.

The therapist's understanding of the stressors that affect Dominican immigrants helped her develop her role as a culture broker for Mr. D and to explain the acculturation process and its accompanying features to him. She was able to help Mr. D integrate aspects of the new culture while retaining the healthy aspects of the former. Therapeutic intervention helped to prevent marital separation and other problems such as domestic violence, substance abuse, and worsening psychiatric distress, such as depression, which often results from situations like this one. Recognizing the need for therapy and providing early intervention give families the opportunity to successfully work through some of the painful stresses that can accompany acculturation.

REFERENCES

Bosch J: Composiciòn Social Dominicana: Historìa e Interpretaciòn, 14th Edition. Santo Domingo, Republica Dominicana, Alfa y Omega, 1984

Bray DB: The Dominican exodus: origins, problems, solutions, in The Caribbean Exodus. Edited by Levine BB. New York, Praeger, 1987, pp 152–171

Consejo Nacional de Educación Superior (CONES): About CONES. Available at: http://www.cones.gov.do

Cosgrove J: Remigration: the Dominican experience. Social Development Issues 14:213, 1992

Gil RM, Vazquez CI: The Maria Paradox: How Latinas Can Merge Old World Traditions With New World Self-Esteem. New York, GP Putnam's Sons, 1996

Moya Pons F: Manual de Historìa Dominicana, Vol 9. Santiago, Dominican Republic, Universidad Catòlica Madre y Maestra, 1984

Pellerano & Herrera (attorneys): A Lawyer's Guide to the Dominican Republic. Santo Domingo, Republica Dominicana, Lex Mundi, 2001. Available at: http://www.hg.org/guide-domrep.html

Plan Nacional de Salud Mental. Santo Domingo, Republica Dominicana, 2000

Rodriguez O, Cooney SR, Gilberson G, et al: Nuestra Amèrica en Nueva York: The New Immigrant Hispanic Populations in New York City 1980–1990. New York, The Hispanic Research Center, Fordham University, 1995

Tejada Ortiz D, Sanchez-Martinez F, Rejias-Mella C: Religiosidad Popular y Psiquiatría. Santo Domingo, Republica Dominicana, Editora Corripio, C por A, 1993

Urena HM: Panorama Històrico de la Literatura Dominicana, 2nd Edition. Santo Domingo, Republica Dominicana, Coleccion Pensamiento, 1966

Wiarda JA: The Dominican Republic: A Nation in Transition. New York, Praeger, 1969

Zaglul A: Prologo, in Religiosidad Popular y Psiquiatría. Santo Domingo, Republica Dominicana, Editora Corripio, C por A, 1993

CHAPTER 7

Salvadorans

Carlos B. Cordova, Ed.D.
Felix Kury, M.A.

EL SALVADOR, A TROPICAL land of lakes, valleys, and volcanoes, is the smallest country in the Americas. Located in Central America, it is bordered by Guatemala to the northwest, Honduras to the northeast, and the Pacific Ocean to the west. It is about the size of the state of Massachusetts, with 8,260 square miles.

According to demographic data of 1995, El Salvador has a population of 5,769,000. This is one of the highest densities in the world—about 698 persons per square mile. Overall, the Salvadoran population is young: 40.7% are under 15 years of age, and only 6.2% are over 60.

About 85% of the population are *mestizos*, or people of mixed Indian and Spanish blood. Only 10% of the people are Indian. Most Salvadorans are Roman Catholics, but they retain ancient indigenous cultural and religious traditions that have been syncretized with European beliefs. During recent decades other religious denominations such as Baptist and Lutheran have gained popularity.

El Salvador has one of the most skewed socioeconomic systems in Latin America. Huge gaps exist between social classes, and there are marked inequities between rich and poor. It is estimated that about 300 families (2% of the population) control most of the nation's wealth. There is a small middle class composed of professionals and entrepreneurs, but the great majority of the population lives in poverty. The unemployment rate in 1995 was 7.5%. Most employed persons held jobs that paid subsistence wages.

Since the 1950s, El Salvador has attempted to industrialize its economy. The government has approved policies that attracted assembly-line industry and promoted economic growth. Unfortunately, this form of economic development has benefited only the small power elite; the majority of population only provides the labor and is underpaid. The creation of these urban industries has stimulated migration from rural areas to the capital city, San Salvador, where factories and industrial plants are located.

It is estimated that in the 1960s, 70% of the population lived in rural areas. By 1995, only 52.1% remained in rural areas and 47.9% resided in urban communities. Rural people exhibit low levels of education and usually work in agricultural activities such as farm labor. The urban experience is new for most Salvadorans. Significant proportions belong to the lower levels of the urban class structure and live in poor neighborhoods and marginal communities. The majority work as laborers in assembly-line factories. The influx of workers into the cities has been greater than the actual need for labor, and serious problems have surfaced in urban areas in housing, health care, crime, employment, and social stability.

THE SALVADORAN CIVIL WAR

Between 1979 and 1992, El Salvador experienced a cruel and violent civil war. The generalized state of fear and anguish experienced by Salvadorans as a result of the repression of the period plays an important role in the cultural and social framework of the Salvadoran people.

During the late 1970s, government forces silenced selected religious, student, and labor leaders through torture or murder. In the early 1980s the strategy of the war changed from selective repression to a general conflict that involved the entire population. The long-term effect of the war was the erosion of the country's social fabric and the destruction of individual lives, as exemplified by the breakdown of trust, security, and solidarity.

The war left more than 75,000 people dead, and over 9,000 had disappeared. Most of these people were noncombatants killed in military missions carried out by the Salvadoran army and its paramilitary forces. Both military groups received financial assistance from the United States. The arbitrary detention or abduction of a person, followed by disappearance, became a common practice of the security forces in the Latin American countries governed under the Doctrine of National Security (Dussin 1986). In El Salvador this tactic had the objectives of both eliminating the "subversive" and instilling terror in his or her family and neighbors with the use of irregular forces, such as death squads. The uncertainty of who would be the next victim served to give the general impression of absolute control and impunity.

Over 1 million people, about 20% of Salvadorans, were forcibly moved from their communities and homeland. Approximately 600,000 *campesinos* (farm laborers) became refugees within their own country. Another 800,000 people sought refuge in the United States, Canada, Mexico, other Central American countries, and places as far away as Australia (American Civil Liberties Union 1984; Camarda 1985, Cordova 1987, 1995a, 1995b; Kury 1987).

HISTORY OF MIGRATION TO THE UNITED STATES

Salvadorans have migrated to the United States since the early 1900s. They have relocated as a result of the political and economic factors that have historically affected their country. The early immigrants came during the 1930s and 1940s, resettling in San Francisco, Los Angeles, Houston, and New Orleans. They left El Salvador to escape economic failure and political persecution. These pioneers helped to establish the social and economic foundations of the Latino immigrant community and would provide support to future generations of Salvadorans to arrive in the United States.

During the 1960s, an increase in Salvadoran immigration to the United States can be credited to the Immigration Act of 1965, which granted immigrant quotas to countries that historically had not been included in its immigration policies. The 1965 law encouraged Salvadoran professionals and skilled laborers to migrate to the United States and permitted the resettlement of large numbers of young working-class Salvadoran families. Several cities in the United States had Latin American immigrant neighborhoods, and Salvadorans were attracted to them. By and large, the newcomers resettled in Latino neighborhoods because of already established ethnic networks, familiar cultural traditions, and readily available support systems. The new Salvadoran arrivals helped to further develop the economic, social, and cultural foundations of Latino enclaves in San Francisco, Los Angeles, Houston, New York, and Washington, D.C.

The influx of Salvadorans into the United States has increased sharply since the late 1970s. According to data from the U.S. Bureau of the Census (Montgomery 1994) and the U.S. Immigration and Naturalization Service (1994), there were approximately 625,000 Salvadorans living in the United States in 1993. El Salvador ranks as third among Latin American countries in the number of immigrants it contributes to the United States (Cordova and Rivera-Pinderhughes 1999). However, the numbers are thought to be much higher because these official sources exclude the large numbers of undocumented Salvadorans. Some estimates place the total Salvadoran population in the United States at well over 1 million people (Cordova and Rivera-Pinderhughes 1999).

Before the 1970s most Salvadorans arrived in the United States with permanent resident status or with student visas. In the 1980s, the Salvadoran civil war changed the migration patterns, and large numbers of Salvadorans began to enter the United States without legal documentation or as political asylum applicants. The pre-1979 migration was mostly planned and economic in nature, whereas the post-1979 migrations were generated by both the economic and the political threats faced by the Salvadoran population (American Civil Liberties Union 1984, Cordova 1987, 1995a, 1995b).

MENTAL HEALTH ISSUES OF SALVADORANS

The literature regarding the Salvadoran populations living in the United States is extremely limited. There are only a handful of journal articles and books that provide a comprehensive analysis of the social, cultural, economic, and psychological experiences of this group. Various authors have stressed the importance of researching and documenting information about this group (Cordova 1995b).

In El Salvador it is believed that only the severely mentally ill should consult a psychologist. The general population is not familiar with mental health concepts and psychological treatment. Upon arrival in the United States many Salvadoran immigrants reject recommendations made by their more acculturated relatives and friends who encourage them to seek mental health services. Many immigrants have a variety of problems associated with acculturation, such as anxiety, stress, and depression. Among the undocumented workers there are also high levels of anxiety, depression, and posttraumatic stress stemming from the constant fear of deportation, mistrust of governmental authorities, and their past life experiences.

A variety of models of psychological treatment may be used to work effectively with the Salvadoran populations in the United States. Psychiatric medications are very effective with more severe forms of psychiatric disorders, as are family, individual, and group therapy, school-based counseling, and case management services. We have continuously integrated aspects of Paulo Freire's (1973) critical consciousness teaching models in the development of clinical work with Salvadorans. These critical theories have been effective because they generate reflection and participation on the part of both the client and the clinician. These methodologies have been used to successfully develop and implement support groups and psychoeducational groups and to train health promoters. Protocols have also been developed by which to refer clients undergoing psychiatric crisis episodes to social rehabilitation programs as an alternative to inpatient psychiatric treatment.

IMPACT OF THE CIVIL WAR ON SALVADORAN IMMIGRANTS

The social polarization that still exists in El Salvador as a residual effect of the civil war can also be observed among the communities of Salvadorans in the United States. Martin-Baró's (1989) psychosocial trauma framework states that every Salvadoran has been affected by the war and its generalized climate of violence, without regard to social status, residential patterns, or migration histories. Social trauma is used to refer to the way a historic process can leave an entire population affected. As Martin-Baró would argue,

> This is not to say that some uniform effect is produced throughout the population, or that one can assume the experience of war has some mechanical impact on people.... the injury or damage depends on the particular experience of each individual, an experience conditioned by his or her social background and the degree of participation in the conflict as well as other characteristics of the individual's personality and experience. (Martin-Baró 1989, p. 10)

To those not familiar with the Salvadoran conflict, it may sound like an overstatement when claims are made that every Salvadoran family had a relative die as a direct result of the general conditions of the war. All Salvadorans have been deeply affected by the war; these effects are rooted in each individual's involvement in the conflict, area of residence, occupation, and family relations.

It is important to note that the events occurring in El Salvador continue to have a deep and serious impact on Salvadoran populations living abroad. These events can be social, cultural, political, or economic. For example, at the time of the 1986 earthquake in San Salvador, many working-class communities were leveled by seismic activity, leaving many people dead and wounded. The impact of the earthquake severely affected Salvadoran communities throughout the world as the immigrants worried about their relatives and friends and had difficulty obtaining enough news about what was occurring in the country. A high incidence of emotional trauma and psychological crises was reported in Salvadoran communities throughout the United States during this period.

Another example of this type of emotional trauma was felt during the 1989 Frente Farabundo Martí para la Liberación Nacional (FMLN) offensive against the government. At that time the left carried out a military campaign throughout El Salvador, affecting the capital for the first time. Working-class communities were bombed by the Salvadoran air force, and many people were left dead or wounded. The details of the episode were slow to reach the United States, and the names of the dead and wounded did not arrive for several days. A crisis developed in Salvadoran immigrant communities in the United States, and many people begin to manifest a variety of psychiatric symptoms such as anxiety, depression, chest pains, and guilt about being unable to attend the funerals.

Many immigrants continue to manifest symptoms of trauma secondary to the war and continuing crises in El Salvador for many years, as is illustrated in this case example:

Mr. and Mrs. E and their children left El Salvador and came to the United States in 1980 after the war there became increasingly repressive. Previously, they had visited this country frequently, because they had two other children who had been living in San Francisco since the 1960s. Two days after their arrival, men wearing green uniforms assassinated Mrs. E's brother in El Salvador. When she learned of her brother's death and realized she could not return to his funeral and take part in the traditional bereavement ceremonies, she began to manifest emotional distress and a wide range of psychosomatic problems such as muscular and chest pains, anxiety, and depression.

In 1986, after the earthquake in San Salvador, the family learned that the house where the family business was located had been destroyed, and Mr. E became seriously worried about the fate of a son living still living in San Salvador. Mr. E suffered a massive stroke and was hospitalized for 6 months. He was brought home, and Mrs. E cared for him for 2 years, until her own health begin to decline and the doctors stated that her condition would only worsen if she continued to care for her husband. She did not want to place him a convalescent home because she saw this as a breach of tradition and family responsibility. Finally, after counseling and several family meetings, with the support of her family she agreed to have him placed. She continued to visit Mr. E daily, and they both responded well to the move.

Mrs. E, however, continued to worry about her oldest son, who was still living in El Salvador. He had to travel every day through areas that were affected by the political strife, and on several occasions he was caught in the cross fire between the government and guerrillas. Mrs. E's anxiety and depression increased because of her inability to be with her son and his refusal to come to the United States. In 1989, during the FMLN offensive, she had a major psychiatric crisis. When U.S. television news reports showed airplanes attacking the neighborhood where her son lived, she developed severe anxiety attacks and chest pains and was hospitalized in a medical unit for

3 days. In the early 1990s, when her symptoms still had not improved and continued to increase, her doctors finally recommended that she seek mental health treatment. She refused to do so for a long time, but finally in 1992 her children persuaded her to seek the help of psychologists. With time, Mrs. E's symptoms decreased and she became less dependent on her medications. She participated more in social activities and even joined a local senior citizen's center. In 1994, when Mr. E died, she was able to prepare for the moment with the support of the therapist and family members; she went through all the funeral ceremonies and coped with the situation well. As of the time of this writing, she was doing quite well and had adjusted to her new life in the United States.

PSYCHOLOGICAL CONSEQUENCES OF WAR TRAUMA

Individuals who themselves were victims or whose family members were victims of the political violence in El Salvador frequently manifest various forms of psychological problems after arrival and settlement in the United States. Victims of torture often have the symptoms of posttraumatic stress disorder (PTSD). They include severe depression, guilt, nightmares, flashbacks, hyperalertness, insomnia, suicidal tendencies, and withdrawal. The psychiatric evaluation of Central Americans conducted at refugee centers throughout the San Francisco Bay area concluded that a large number of people there suffered from PTSD (Cordova 1987).

There are common characteristics observed in Salvadoran immigrants, refugees, and undocumented workers. They often migrate alone and have few relatives or friends in the host society. There is often a sudden disruption in the relationship with the family and homeland, which can be severely distressing. Involuntary sudden departure does not allow for saying goodbye or for making preparations to leave. Many of these immigrants often find themselves reliving past experiences in El Salvador to the point of becoming obsessed and disturbed. Sometimes their solitude and their recurring memories give rise to suicidal moods.

Many of these immigrants are undocumented in the United States and live in fear of being apprehended and returned home. Because of the fear of deportation, they often underuse even the medical and social services set up help them. When seen for psychiatric treatment, they are often brought to community clinics or hospitals against their will by family, friends, or—if in acute distress—the police.

To understand the quality and magnitude of what some of these immigrants have experienced, one must envision the extreme cruelty that drenches the most typical act of violence: torture. In El Salvador an environment of fear and distrust was imposed by means of aerial bombings; kidnappings; the killing of priests, nuns, and students; the raping and torturing of women; and the decapitating and dismembering of bodies (Martin-Baró 1983). Such torture breaks the individual's will to struggle and makes him or her unable to find a space in which to reintegrate. Without a context, the individual is forced to flee the community, changing his or her family's aspirations and social realities.

A common practice during the war was the macabre exhibit of mutilated bodies scattered on sidewalks or thrown into garbage dumps—such horrors as mothers with their wombs ripped open and the fetuses cut up. It was also common to see headless bodies hung from school halls or tree branches and labeled "enemies of public order" on papers signed by the death squads (Martin-Baró 1983). It is within this dimension of personal suffering that one begins to understand how families eager to find their relatives were unable to identify them publicly when they found them. In silence and sorrow, they removed themselves from these scenes, only to have their pain internalized and negated. They dissociated themselves from the reality around them and developed silence as both a symptom of suffering and a mechanism of survival. A common example of this negation was the transformation of language to euphemize the terror by simply describing the war or war-related events as "la situacìon" (the situation) (Cordova 1987).

Rape, concomitant with torture, was probably the most prevalent form of sexual abuse committed against women captured by the Salvadoran military. Commonly, women were sodomized or subjected to electroshock in their nipples and vaginas. It was common in war zones for a young woman to "voluntarily" allow herself to be "protected" by an individual soldier to avoid becoming the property of a whole battalion (Martin-Baró 1989).

Salvadoran refugees in the United States who are survivors of the experiences described above manifested the same psychiatric symptoms as their counterparts who remained in El Salvador. This case exemplifies the varying degrees of damage caused by those social conditions and treatment outcomes.

> Ms. F, a 28-year-old woman, sought psychiatric treatment after she began to experience insomnia, recurring dreams of past traumatic events, and the inability to concentrate. She had been living in the San Francisco Bay area for a brief period and was a domestic worker. Her children were scheduled to arrive from El Salvador soon, and she feared that her condition was going to deteriorate and she would be unable to care for them.
>
> Ms. F's history revealed that in 1988, while living in El Salvador, she had been abducted by the National Guard. Even though she was not an activist, she was arrested because she was the sister of a labor leader accused of being a rebel in the FMLN, the guerrilla force in El Salvador.

During therapy Ms. F was able to recount the details of her captivity. She recalled that soldiers came to her house, forced her into a truck, and then kept her imprisoned for a total of 5 months. During the early days of her captivity she was kept blindfolded; stripped naked, raped, and tortured by as many as 10 guards. She painfully remembered the day a lieutenant came to her cell and offered to protect her from the abuse of the other men. A week after being released from her ordeal, she was finally able to leave the country with the support of a human rights organization.

Ms. F received her treatment at a psychiatric residential treatment center after another refugee had referred her there. In the initial stage of treatment, the treating staff's goal was to develop a nurturing environment for her so that her trust could be gained. When she finally begin to tell her story, she felt great shame and anger because she had accepted protection from a government official to avoid mass rape. She had difficulty acknowledging that she had been in an extremely difficult position where her options were severely limited—either allowing herself to be raped by one officer or continuing to be subjected to mass rape.

In the treatment Ms. F was helped to reframe her experience: that she was a survivor rather than a victim of torture and other traumatic events. She eventually managed to learn how to live with her trauma and is now leading a productive life. She has gained a sense of purpose, identity, and belonging through her work in solidarity groups and in her participation in antiwar efforts and fund-raising for humanitarian aid to El Salvador.

She also learned to find solace and healing within the refugee and solidarity community. She found her association with these groups to offer more therapeutic relief than did the mental health agencies in the community. Ms. F participated in weekly meetings, vigils, religious ceremonies, and other assemblies. She, like other refugees, found it therapeutic to be with people who understood her plight and provided spiritual comfort.

In working with clients like Ms. F, it is important to evaluate what agencies will provide the best treatment. Some people find contacts with the mental health system of the United States to be traumatic, particularly when they are brought into involuntary treatment. Outpatient treatment can also be difficult if the therapist is insensitive to the state of the client and either pushes for information about torture and other traumatic events too fast or ignores them completely.

Some clients, like Ms. F, find that solidarity committees are helpful and therapeutic. In this setting, where people understand the experiences of the survivor, people learn to restructure their behavior patterns, and they are allowed to integrate their experiences of loss and to establish the truth of what happened to them. The ending of silence and denial allows people to confront their pain as well as the myth that not speaking of one's pain will make it go away. In these settings, survivors develop an awareness that their individual suffering is intimately connected to the social suffering experienced by all Salvadorans and that individual illnesses are nothing more than metaphors of social destruction (Lira 1989).

The referral of refugees to solidarity committees rather than mental health clinics has been a controversial issue. There is a question on the part of some professionals about the validity and therapeutic nature of these group activities. Some clinicians argue that encouraging clients to become involved in political work supports clients' delusional systems and feelings of grandiosity. It is our observation, however, that some individuals who were labeled as sick or as mental health patients eventually went on to become mental health clients with chronic conditions. In saying this, one has to be careful not to generalize that all contacts with the mental health system are toxic or that all experiences with refugee or solidarity committees are therapeutic. Each case must be considered from the viewpoint of the client's symptoms, his or her plight, and what the client sees as providing him or her with therapeutic relief. As in the case of Ms. F, sometimes a connection with both systems of care can be successfully integrated.

TREATMENT RECOMMENDATIONS FOR INTERVENTION WITH SALVADORANS

Healing the pain of migration, violence, and war is a difficult task. Salvadorans may not be familiar with the individually based approaches of mental health treatment as practiced in the United States and may continue to seek support from family. They may also hold the belief that healthy, sane persons do not seek the services of psychiatrists or other mental health providers—that only the crazy or severely mentally ill do so.

The following recommendations will help to engage people in treatment:

- A variety of treatment models may be used when dealing with Salvadoran populations in the United States, and each person must be evaluated to determine which is the most appropriate for him or her.
- Clinicians working with Salvadorans must have an understanding of Salvadoran cultural patterns as well as of the sociopolitical issues affecting this immigrant population.
- It is important to develop protocols to be used in referring clients undergoing a psychiatric crisis. The integration of traditional treatment in social rehabilitation programs with community-based support groups, psychoeducational groups, and support by health providers may in some cases provide the best treatment outcomes.

REFERENCES

American Civil Liberties Union: Salvadorans in the United States: The Case for Extended Voluntary Departure (National Immigration and Alien Rights Project Report No 1). Washington, DC, American Civil Liberties Union, April 1984

Camarda R: Forced to Move: Salvadoran Refugees in Honduras. San Francisco, CA, Solidarity Publications, 1985

Cordova CB: Undocumented El Salvadorans in the San Francisco Bay area: migration and adaptation dynamics. Journal of La Raza Studies 1(1):9–37, 1987

Cordova CB: The social, cultural and religious experiences of Central American immigrants in the United States, in Dialogue Rejoined: Theology and Ministry in the United States Hispanic Reality. Edited by Pineada AM, Schreiter R. Collegeville, MN, Liturgical Press, 1995a, pp 23–42

Cordova CB: Organizing in Central American immigrant communities in the United States (Chapter 10), in Community Organizing in a Diverse Society, 2nd Edition. Edited by Rivera FG, Erlich JL. Boston, MA, Allyn & Bacon, 1995b

Cordova CB, Rivera-Pinderhughes R: Central and South Americans (Chapter 5), in A Nation of Peoples: A Sourcebook on America's Multicultural Heritage. Edited by Barkan ER. Westport, CT, Greenwood Press, 1999

Dussin J: Torture in Brazil. New York, Random House, 1986

Freire P: Education for Critical Consciousness. New York, NY, Seabury Press, 1973

Kury FS: Torture syndrome as a specific case of post-traumatic stress disorder in Salvadoran refugees. Journal of La Raza Studies 1(1):38–42, 1987

Lira E: Daño social y memoria colectiva: perspectiva de reparaciòn, derechos humanos: todo es segùn ed dolor con que se mira. Santiago, Chile, Instituto Latinoamericano de Salud Mental y Derechos Humanos (ILAS), Maturana, 1989

Martin-Baró I: Acciòn e Ideologìa: Psicologìa social desde Centroamerica. San Salvador, El Salvador, Universidad Centroamericana, 1983

Martin-Baró I: Political violence and war as causes of psychosocial trauma in El Salvador. Journal of La Raza Studies 2(2):5–15, 1989

Montgomery PA: The Hispanic Population in the United States: March 1993. Current Population Reports, Series P-20: Population Characteristics, No. 475. Washington, DC, U.S. Bureau of the Census, June 1994

U.S. Immigration and Naturalization Service: 1993 Statistical Yearbook of the Immigration and Naturalization Service. Washington, DC, U.S. Government Printing Office, 1994

CHAPTER 8

Mexicans

Cervando Martinez Jr., M.D.

THE PEOPLE OF MEXICAN descent in the United States are similar to other immigrant groups from Latin America in many ways—language, religion, and general cultural characteristics. They also differ in one significant way: most are not recent immigrants. Although many are recent arrivals in the United States, many more are multigenerational Californians or Tejanos (Texans of Mexican ancestry). In fact, many Hispanics in New Mexico connect themselves much more with the Spanish settlers of that region than with any Mexican heritage. In south Texas it is not unusual to find Mexican Americans who speak predominantly Spanish and are very Mexican in some of their habits, yet have difficulty identifying any specific family connection to Mexico. They may even, among friends, call themselves *mejicanos,* but they have no immediate relatives in Mexico and have never traveled there and do not expect to do so. Thus, a clinician treating Mexican Americans is confronted by a wide range of individuals who may differ quite remarkably in language use, acculturation, and ethnic identification. This wide range of ethnic types among Mexican Americans has been described in detail elsewhere (Keefe and Padilla 1987). Nevertheless, it is of importance to have some understanding of Mexico to understand Mexican Americans, because whether or not a Mexican American acknowledges a cultural debt to Mexico, the influence of this country, especially in the southwestern states, cannot be ignored.

Mexico is virtually next door, with its densely populated border cities pushing against their small United States counterparts. The movement of people back and forth across the 2,000-mile border is massive and includes large numbers of persons who travel one way or the other for medical or dental care, medications, or other health-related purposes. Many Americans cross into Mexico for less expensive medical and dental care, whereas Mexicans may cross into the United States for more expensive but presumably better quality medical care. Many Americans obtain their prescription drugs in Mexico, where they are more readily available and cheaper. These patterns can result in problems of discontinuity of care, abuse of prescription medications—particularly amphetamines and benzodiazepines—and the development of antibiotic-resistant infections. Many pregnant Mexican women cross the border to give birth in order to give their children United States citizenship.

Mexico itself is a vast and heterogeneous country. The northern tier of states (Nuevo Leon, Chihuahua, Baja California) are more prosperous than most of the central states (Guanajuato, Michoacan) or the southern states (Chiapas, Oaxaca). When immigrating to the United States, Mexicans usually follow established village or town patterns, settling where other people from their community already live in large numbers; others follow friends and relatives. The availability of jobs in a particular United States community is also a powerful factor. During times of United States economic recession, immigration from Mexico slows down and in some cases reverses itself as people return to Mexico.

The Mexican people themselves are diverse, ranging from the somewhat Americanized *norteños* (northerners) to the urban *capitalinos* (residents of Mexico City), to the villagers of all of Mexico, to the indigenous (Indian) population of the southern states. The indigenous people, although not restricted to the southern states, often still speak a native language plus Spanish. In recent years, they have drawn international attention to their many social and economic problems by their revolt in Chiapas.

Although the stereotypical Mexican immigrant to the United States may be a young man or woman with limited education from a small town or village in one of the poor states of Mexico, this picture is certainly not reflective of the general population of Mexico, which may be more urban, educated, and employed. As has occurred in the United States, the population of Mexico has become increasingly urban; cities that have experienced a large amount of growth include Mexico City, Guadalajara, Monterey, Tijuana, and Cuidad Juarez. At the time of this writing, 68% of the Mexican population lived in a community with more than 2,000 inhabitants.

Although all Latin American countries have a historical relationship with the United States, the United States–Mexico relationship is probably the most extensive and complex. At the heart of the relationship is the fact that a large portion of the United States once belonged to Mexico and was "won" by the United States in the Mexican War of the last century. During the preceding centuries, the Southwest region of the present-day United States constituted the northern provinces of colonial Spain and was settled by means of missions and forts, first by Spaniards and later by Mexicans. Early settlers intermarried with the Native Americans and later with the western-migrating white settlers. The descendants of these early Spanish colonists and Native American and white settlers had become the native population of the Southwest at the time of the Mexican War. After the war, American settlement and takeover of previously Mexican property and institutions accelerated, and the relative number of natives declined (Montejano 1987). However, migration from Mexico continued and then accelerated during and after the Mexican Revolution of 1910.

The events of the Mexican historical legacy have resulted in the development of an ambivalent attitude by Mexicans toward the United States. On the one hand, the historical legacy of war, loss of territory, interference in internal affairs, economic domination, and racist attitudes of many Americans toward Mexicans have resulted in the negative aspect of Mexicans' attitudes toward the United States. Admiration for and attraction to American progress, power, and wealth pull in the opposite direction.

HEALTH CARE IN MEXICO

The Mexican American has usually had little contact with the Mexican health care system in general and much less with its mental health component. The recent Mexican immigrant, on the other hand, has probably had some contact with the Mexican health care system, particularly its public health and primary care facilities. The Mexican health care system consists of several federal systems, limited local facilities (*hospitales civiles*), and a private sector. The public sector makes up approximately 90% of the system. The public system is organized by primary, secondary, and tertiary care facilities and includes community-based primary care urban and rural clinics and specialty clinics; tertiary facilities are often affiliated with medical schools. The system offers a wide range of services, from the most rudimentary public health to sophisticated interventions comparable to any in the world.

Mental health services are limited to the larger cities and consist of outpatient psychiatric clinics in general regional hospitals, inpatient units in the larger medical centers, and *hospitales granjas*, long-term facilities similar to the older state hospitals in the United States. The private psychiatric systems consist of freestanding hospitals or inpatient units of general hospitals.

Mexico has approximately 1,000 psychiatrists. Clinical psychologists, many without a doctorate, function as therapists in both the private and the public sector. Social workers are not trained to provide psychotherapy. Psychoanalysis has had a strong influence on the theoretic orientation of psychiatrists and psychologists. Some analytic schools of thought, such as those of Klein and Fromm, have had greater relative influence in Mexico than in the United States. However, in recent years the influence of biological psychiatry has been increasingly dominant in the Mexican psychiatric training programs.

- Because Mexican immigrants to the United States are more likely to be young men and women from small or rural communities, psychiatric services may not have been available to them in Mexico, even if they have experienced psychiatric symptoms. Their attitudes about mental illness may parallel those of rural working-class people in other countries:
- Mental illness is believed to be caused by a combination of stressful life events, bad experiences, genes, supernatural factors, and factors that are part of folk beliefs (hex, soul loss).
- Treatment is not sought until the condition is intolerable to the family; prior to that, a variety of other measures are taken, such as advice from friends and relatives, folk remedies, symptomatic relief from a pharmacist or primary care clinic, or spiritual intervention. (In particular, specific requests are made to Catholic saints, sometimes by making pilgrimages to the saint's home church.)

The nature of Mexican populations influences the distribution of mental disorders. Because the population tends to be younger, the mental health problems of children and young people tend to assume greater relative significance. Services for children and families are provided through a distinct multidisciplinary system, the Centros de Integración Juvenil, a federal network of state-based social service programs, which include mental health services for children and families. The major psychiatric disorders (e.g., schizophrenia, affective disorders) occur at rates similar to those in other countries, including the United States; however, there are significant dissimilarities in patterns of drug and alcohol use and abuse.

PATTERNS OF SUBSTANCE USE AND ABUSE

Alcohol and tobacco are the two substances most abused in Mexico. However, the rate of abstinence from alcohol is higher in Mexican women than in U.S. women (58%–84%, depending on age, probably because of more traditional attitudes and customs). Mexico does not have a heroin problem of the magnitude found in the United States, and cocaine addiction is not as prevalent as in the United States, although clusters of increased use of these two substances have been seen in some northern Mexican cities and in Mexico City (Medina-Mora et al. 1989). Furthermore, the abuse of volatile substances (inhalants), most commonly thinners of different types, is an extremely important problem in Mexican urban adolescent males (Medina-Mora and Berenzon 1995).

Gilbert (1986) described patterns of alcohol consumption and abuse in Mexico and the United States. The prototypical Mexican pattern of consumption is that of intermittent high-volume consumption in men. The typical United States pattern is that of frequent (perhaps daily) low-volume consumption (i.e., the cocktail before dinner pattern). Among Mexican Americans, a blending of the United States with the Mexican pattern appears to occur, resulting in a tendency among Mexican American men to drink more and on a daily basis. The high abstention rates among Mexican American women are maintained but are not as high as those in Mexico.

CLINICAL CONSIDERATIONS

Clinical work with Mexican Americans requires a considerable amount of flexibility by the therapist and the system providing mental health care. This is because of the wide range of acculturation and Spanish language dominance among Mexican Americans. At one extreme are those who are almost completely acculturated and assimilated and may speak little or no Spanish. In some United States communities, this may be a significantly large group, particularly among young adults. The patients may not present the clinician with the challenge of delivering care in the Spanish language or with the appropriate cultural nuance, but issues of culture and language still may be very relevant in therapy. In this situation, the patient may have troublesome issues as a result of not being fluent in Spanish or feeling disconnected from a cultural base or heritage. It is not, of course, invariable that a highly acculturated Mexican American will have conflict about not speaking Spanish; many have resolved this conflict, but many have not, and, thus, it may represent a significant issue at some time in the therapy. Similarly, such individuals may continue to harbor traditional attitudes or beliefs that they act on or that result in conflict with other beliefs. Noteworthy are attitudes toward gender roles and family relationships. A very acculturated Mexican American may yearn for the more traditional family relationships yet consider other aspects of the culture as "old fashioned."

At the other extreme is the immigrant who speaks almost no English and also retains full Mexican cultural baggage. The principal challenge with this patient, in addition to the usual clinical ones, has to do with adequate communication. A large proportion of Mexican Americans (more than 60%) report speaking predominantly Spanish at home (Grebler et al. 1970). Adequate communication with a patient who speaks little or no English may require the use of a translator or the availability of sufficient Spanish-speaking personnel. Acosta and Cristo (1981) reported the successful use of interpreters with Spanish-speaking patients in mental health settings. Providing sufficient Spanish-speaking personnel in a mental health service program, whether private or public, may not be feasible in many communities, especially those with rapidly growing Hispanic immigrant populations and relatively few native Hispanics (e.g., Houston, Texas).

Assessment of a patient's acculturation level helps the clinician evaluate how strongly the patient adheres to traditional Latino values and customs, which might affect clinical behavior. Although several acculturation scales have been developed (Rogler et al. 1991), language use and, to a lesser extent, generation in the United States can be used as surrogates for acculturation. This is a difficult area to evaluate because some individuals and families make conscious attempts to take on United States customs and values, perhaps driven by a need to blend into this society or because of a personal need to reject their Mexican origin. However, many, especially the more recent immigrants, maintain their strong sense of loyalty to many traditional customs and values, while absorbing some United States values.

FAMILY RELATIONSHIPS

Strong evidence indicates that Mexican Americans, as a group, tend to maintain traditional values about the role of the family in life (Montiel 1973). This evidence includes population figures that show higher numbers of intact families and focused studies that show continued allegiance to specific values. Among the areas that merit assessment are

- Role and status of the patient within the family and accompanying expectations (e.g., caring for parents in their older years or for younger siblings)
- Role of nuclear and extended family (the extent to which the extended family is helpful/supportive, distant/unavailable, or problematic to the individual patient)
- Family issues that significantly influence the patient's development and current life functioning (unresolved family grief, family secrets, family disruption)

- Intergenerational conflict, which is of particular significance to more recently immigrated families when children rapidly acquire United States values (including loss of Spanish language fluency, perceived lack of respect for parents and elders, and dating behavior)

TRADITIONAL HEALTH BELIEFS

Many Mexicans and Mexican Americans continue to adhere to traditional beliefs and practices about health and illnesses. Martinez (1977) described these beliefs and their relevance to psychiatric diagnosis. It is important that clinicians have some awareness of the existence of these beliefs, particularly *mal puesto* (hex), because of its common occurrence and potential for influencing the clinical process. Some Mexican American patients and/or their families may conclude that a mental disorder was caused by a hex placed on the patient by another person who has reason to be jealous of the patient. Although it is not known how often this belief occurs in relation to mental illness, some studies reported a 66% rate of knowledge of the condition and a 30% rate of having either experienced the condition personally or had it occur in an immediate family member (Martinez and Martin 1966). It is important to determine whether any elements of this belief complex are actively held by the patient or family for the following reasons: 1) a folk healer (*curandero* or *curandera*) may be consulted in addition to the mental health professional; 2) although the *curandero* usually does not interfere with the health professional, it is important to know what has been or is being recommended as an alternative; and 3) even though in most cases the patient and family comfortably believe in and use both systems, in rare cases the belief in the hex is held in an almost delusional way to avoid dealing with the even more painful reality of possible mental illness.

The use of traditional herbal preparations in Mexican and Mexican Americans is also very extensive, and several of these are prescribed for *nervios* (nerves), sexual problems, anger, and other life problems. Of note is the recent emergence of *uña de gato* (cat's claw), an herbal preparation from Mexico very commonly sold for a variety of conditions.

COMMON EXPRESSIONS OF DISTRESS, ATTITUDES, AND REACTIONS

Mexican Americans express or manifest mental distress or attempt to explain it in a variety of ways. In expressing the most immediate distress, subjective state, or symptom, the expression *nervios* or *estoy nervioso* or *nerviosa* (I am nervous) is probably the most commonly used chief complaint irrespective of eventual underlying disorders. This idiom of distress has been reported in other parts of Latin America and is described extensively by Low (1985). In my experience, this is a neutral phase used to express subjective discomfort regardless of whether the discomfort stems from anxiety, depression, or psychosis. Other phrases are occasionally used, such as *ancioso* (anxious), *desganado* (lacking interest or energy), and *como si quiero correr* (I feel like running—agitation). Nervioso or nerviosa is neutral in the sense that it suggests an emotional problem but does not necessarily imply mental illness (*enfermo mental*) or worse still, *locura* (psychosis or craziness). It thus makes it easier for the person to accept the patient role and the need for treatment.

In attempting to understand the etiology or origin of their disorder, many Mexican Americans elaborate a biopsychosocial explanation that may include family and genetic aspects, intrauterine factors (maternal stress, maternal folk illness, or medical complications), childhood stress (physical or sexual abuse), drug and alcohol abuse, medical disorders, interpersonal conflict, unacceptable or harmful emotions (*coraje,* or anger), and supernatural forces (hexes, the will or punishment by God). It is important to elicit the patient's (and family's) explanation of the problem to more specifically target educational, psychotherapeutic, and even pharmacotherapeutic interventions and to overcome resistance, understand denial, relieve guilt, properly time insight, and avoid excessively painful areas.

SPECIFIC CLINICAL PATTERNS

Several specific psychopathological patterns are commonly observed clinically. Some have also been systematically observed in other Hispanics. Others have not and are more anecdotal. Escobar (1987) described the tendency to somatize in Hispanics, and this certainly occurs in Mexican Americans; however, no evidence, clinical or epidemiologic, suggests greater occurrence in the latter group than in other Hispanics. Anecdotally, the occurrence of mild psychotic symptoms accompanying depressive disorders should be mentioned. These symptoms may consist of fleeting shadows or *bultos* (forms) that occur in the evening and usually are frightening to the patient. They often subside with treatment of the underlying depression or agitation and may not require the administration of antipsychotic medication. The content of delusions may reflect elements of Mexican or Mexican American culture. The *Virgen de Guadalupe,* the patron saint of Mexico, may figure dominantly in religious delusions, as might other cultural entities (e.g., the Mexican mafia and the recently murdered singer Selena Quintanilla). *Ataques de nervios,* often described among

Puerto Ricans (Guarnaccia et al. 1989), have not been observed or reported in Mexican Americans (see Chapter 11 for a complete description of *ataques de nervios*).

ATTITUDES TOWARD PSYCHOTROPIC MEDICATIONS

As suggested earlier in this chapter, Mexican American attitudes toward mental illness reflect a broad underlying perspective encompassing biological to spiritual factors. This perspective is very congruent with psychiatry's biopsychosocial model and thus generally accepting of clinical interpretations or educational feedback about the cause, manifestation, or treatment of a disorder. Thus, acceptance of treatment recommendations, including the use of psychotropic medications, generally is good. Nonetheless, several commonly observed notions about medications should be mentioned. The first, and not necessarily most common, is that many patients are concerned about the addictive potential of all psychotropic medications and about potential problems of psychological dependence. Many Mexican Americans intuitively sense the distinction between physical and psychological dependence but do not have a clear understanding of the potential of psychotropics to result in either of these. Therefore, elucidating this area is often necessary and the results helpful. To date, no evidence indicates that Hispanics require lower dosing or have higher sensitivity to psychotropic medication than do other ethnic groups (Mendoza et al. 1991).

Related to this concern is the worry that taking too many pills at the same time during the day may result in toxic effects or poisoning. This belief also is usually amenable to clarification. These attitudes, of course, do coexist with the individual idiosyncratic attitudes and can result in confusion and poor compliance. However, compliance with medications is increased when these issues are adequately clarified.

The following case example illustrates not only some of the cultural and language barriers that may be encountered when working with Mexican American patients but also how difficult it is to generalize about any cultural group. The case also emphasizes the importance of providing a clinical service that is sensitive to the cultural and language nuances of Mexican Americans.

> Ms. G, a 40-year-old, married, United States–born Mexican American woman, was referred to the Spanish Clinic of the Psychiatry Service operated by the Gynecology Outpatient Service. She was referred because her behavior was quite disturbed and did not permit adequate treatment. On arrival at the clinic, she and her husband loudly demanded the help of a Spanish-speaking psychiatrist. After a brief explanation by the Mexican American at-

tending psychiatrist, a soft-spoken, gentle, Peruvian-born female third-year medical student assessed the patient.

Ms. G related a complex life history that included lifelong physical and sexual abuse that started with her own family, prostitution during her adolescent years, lack of education, polysubstance abuse, marginal work as a barmaid, multiple abusive relationships, recurrent pelvic infections (including treated syphilis), and finally in the last several years a stable relationship with her husband, who was a recovered alcoholic patient with advanced cirrhosis of the liver. The gynecological examinations were being conducted for recurrent pelvic pain and infertility; however, the medical record described several interactions in which Ms. G and her husband became angry with the doctor, and she refused further examination. The notes also reflected anger and frustration on the part of the medical residents (non-Spanish-speaking) attempting to examine her.

Ms. G's psychiatric complaints included a long history of emotional lability, impulsivity, multiple suicidal gestures by wrist slashing, and chronic depression. Recently, she had begun to experience severe insomnia, anger outbursts with her husband, and both auditory and visual (shadows) hallucinations. The auditory hallucinations were loud and condemning.

Her appearance was notable for moderate obesity; childlike petulant demeanor; and multiple tattoos, including the *Pachuco* cross—"t"—on her hands and forehead. She was depressed, irritable, and unable to read or write but was not considered mentally retarded. She described psychotic symptoms, as well as many painful, recurrent, intrusive memories of her traumatic life.

Following the initial assessment and interview with her husband, a mutually agreed-on treatment plan of antidepressant and antipsychotic medications, supportive therapy with the medical student, and facilitation of her return to the Gynecology Outpatient Service for continued care was developed. After several weeks, Ms. G improved symptomatically. Gynecology follow-up was reestablished with the assistance of Spanish-speaking nurses and the social worker, and Ms. G attended the Psychiatry Clinic monthly.

This case is illustrative of

- A United States–born Mexican American patient whose dominant language was Spanish and thus required assessment and therapy in Spanish
- The cultural and language differences between the patient and the gynecological residents, resulting in a breakdown of treatment
- The presence of mild to moderate psychotic symptoms in a person not otherwise thought to have schizophrenia
- An appearance indicative of being part of a Mexican American subculture—the *Pachuco*. (The *Pachucos* were Mexican American young people growing up in the 1940s through 1960s who adopted a unique style of dress, speech, and mannerisms, including the use of the tattoo cross. Some have

described their development as a response to feeling outside of both Mexican and mainstream American cultures, a posture of extreme alienation [Paz 1961].)

•   The fortuitous "match" between a frightened, traumatized woman with many painful and embarrassing memories to share and a gentle, nonthreatening therapist (the medical student) who could be her confidant.

CONCLUSIONS

The above case not only illustrated some of the cultural and language barriers that can be encountered when working with Mexican American patients but also illustrated how difficult it is to generalize about any cultural group. This patient, for example, was extremely alienated from and unsupported by her own family, contrary to the notion that Mexican Americans usually are part of a supportive extended family structure. Nevertheless, the case material also emphasized the importance of providing a clinical service that is sensitive to the cultural and language nuances of this American ethnic group, our nation's second largest. Mexicans in this country and their cousins, the Mexican Americans, will continue to grow in size and importance in the coming decades irrespective of harsher immigration and welfare laws and the dismantling of affirmative action in California and Texas. Thus, American psychiatrists of the future must be knowledgeable about some of the relevant issues in their clinical care. I hope that this brief guide can be useful toward that end.

REFERENCES

Acosta FX, Cristo MH: Development of a bilingual interpreter program: an alternative model for Spanish-speaking services. Professional Psychology: Research and Practice 12:474–482, 1981

Escobar JI: Cross-cultural aspects of the somatization trait. Hospital and Community Psychiatry 38:174–180, 1987

Gilbert J: Alcohol Consumption Among Mexican and Mexican-Americans: A Binational Perspective. Los Angeles, CA, Spanish Speaking Mental Health Research Center, UCLA, 1986

Grebler L, Moore J, Guzman R: The Mexican-American People: The Nation's Second Largest Minority. New York, Free Press, 1970

Guarnaccia PJ, DeLaCancela V, Carrillo E: The multiple meaning of *ataques de nervios* in the Latino community. Med Anthropol 11:47–62, 1989

Keefe SE, Padilla AK: Chicano Ethnicity. Albuquerque, NM, University of New Mexico Press, 1987

Low SM: Culturally interpreted symptoms or culture-bound syndromes: a cross-cultural review of nerves. Soc Sci Med 21:187–196, 1985

Martinez C: Curanderos: clinical aspects. Journal of Operational Psychiatry 8:35–38, 1977

Martinez C, Martin HW: Folk diseases among urban Mexican-Americans. JAMA 196:161–164, 1966

Medina-Mora ME, Berenzon S: Epidemiology of inhalant abuse in Mexico, in Epidemiology of Inhalant Abuse: An International Perspective (NIDA Res Monogr 148; DHHS Publ No NIH 95-3831). Edited by Kozel N, Sloboda Z, De La Rosa M. Washington, DC, U.S. Government Printing Office, 1995, pp 136–174

Medina-Mora ME, Tapia CR, Rascon ML, et al: Situaciòn epidemiològica del abuso de drogas en Mèxico. Bol Oficina Sanit Panam 196:475–484, 1989

Mendoza R, Smith MW, Poland RE, et al: Ethnic psychopharmacology: the Hispanic and Native American perspective. Psychopharmacol Bull 27:449–458, 1991

Montejano D: Anglos and Mexicans in the Making of Texas. Austin, University of Texas Press, 1987

Montiel M: The Chicano family: a review of research. Soc Work 18(2):22–31, 1973

Paz O: The Pachuco and other extremes, in The Labyrinth of Solitude, Life and Thought in Mexico. New York, Grove Press, 1961

Rogler LH, Cortes DE, Malgady RG: Acculturation and Mental Health Status Among Hispanics: Convergence and New Direction for Research. Washington, DC, American Psychological Association, 1991

CHAPTER 9

Nicaraguans

Alvaro LaCayo, M.D.

NICARAGUA IS SITUATED IN the heart of the Americas, Central America. Located between the Pacific Ocean and the Caribbean, Nicaragua is bordered on the south by Costa Rica and on the north by Honduras. The current population of Nicaragua is approximately 4 million people, with 75% of the people being *mestizos* (Spanish and American Indian), followed by 10% European, 11% Creole or African, and 3% indigenous. The country's population is predominantly urban, and most people live in the capital city of Managua. Generally, Nicaragua is a poor country whose economy has continually been devastated by corruption, war, and natural disasters such as earthquakes and hurricanes.

A quarter million Nicaraguans live in the United States. To understand their immigration patterns and their status in this country, it is important to understand the historical factors that have contributed to their lives as exiles and the role that the United States has had in their country's history.

HISTORICAL BACKGROUND

Nicaragua's history can be characterized by its struggle for independence (Bethell 1993; Cuadra 1994; Lainez 1992). Christopher Columbus reached the present-day Central America in 1502 and claimed the area for Spain, but Nicaragua itself was first reached by Gil Gonzalez de Avila in 1522. The Spanish did not develop the economy of the area because it did not produce the gold and silver fortunes they were seeking. The main effect of their settlement was the eradication of the indigenous populations who died as a result of the new diseases that were introduced into the areas and the change from an agrarian economy based on beans, pepper, corn, and cocoa to an economy based on cattle raising.

In 1821, Nicaragua declared independence from Spain and became part of the Mexican Empire under the leadership of General Agustìn de Iturbide. In 1823, to resist Mexico's attempt to control the Central American area, Nicaragua broke away and formed the United Provinces of Central America along with the other Central American states. This union was dissolved in 1837. Another attempt to unite the region as the Greater Republic of Central America failed in 1885, under the leadership of the Ampala Unionist Pact and President Policarpo Bonilla. A later unsuccessful effort to form a federated republic was made in 1921 by Guatemala, Honduras, and El Salvador.

The reason that the unionist fervor never crystallized remains an unsolved enigma. The greed of the local *caudillos* (military dictators) and the separatist influence of foreign countries represent plausible explanations. At a local level, the persistent antagonism of General Francisco Morazan, a pro-unionist liberal executed in 1842, and General Jose Rafael Carrero, a pro-autonomy conservative who died in 1865, probably played a decisive role in this outcome.

The first intervention of the United States military in Nicaragua occurred in the 1850s when William Walker, an American soldier of fortune, attempted to take over the country. The effort to expel him ended up involving all of Central America, the British navy, and the United States marines. In 1909, the marines returned to Nicaragua to help remove Jose Santos Zelaya from power. They remained there until 1925 when the Nicaraguan National Guard was formed, with the assistance of the United States, to maintain order in the country.

Great civil unrest quickly emerged after the marines withdrew until they returned to help prevent civil war in 1927. The struggle during this period saw the emergence of two powerful leaders—Augusto Cesar Sandino and Anastasio Somoza Garcìa—whose influence would forever change the course of Nicaraguan history.

Sandino headed the forces that opposed the United States marines and the Nicaraguan National Guard. This group's efforts were characterized by engaging in guerrilla warfare, primarily in rural areas. In the meantime, when President Herbert Hoover withdrew the marines from Nicaragua in 1933 because of an increasing isolationist sentiment in the United States, Somoza Garcìa was appointed to direct the National Guard. He eventually assumed power over the army and ultimately all of the government. The Somoza era was heralded by the assassination of Sandino in 1934.

Somoza Garcìa remained dictator of Nicaragua for 20 years. During his tenure, he retained a good relationship with the United States and thus continued to receive economic and military aid for his country. When Somoza Garcia was assassinated in 1956, his sons assumed the presidency and control over the National Guard. All the governmental power was concentrated in Anastasio Somoza Debayle in 1967, after his brother had a fatal heart attack.

Somoza Debayle's regime was particularly repressive, and opposition against him led to the end of the Somoza dynasty. Political upheaval escalated after the earthquake of 1972, when the economy dramatically declined. This period saw the emerging influence of the *Frente Sandinista de Liberacìon* (National Liberation Front), which had been formed in the early 1960s. This small university-based group, inspired by Marxist ideology—with Augusto Cesar Sandino as their emblem—and supported by the liberation spirit of the whole of civil society, took over the Nicaraguan government on July 19, 1979.

The United States was not in support of the new government, fearing the emergence of another Cuba. From 1981 to 1989, the Reagan administration authorized financial support for the Contras, a group of former Nicaraguan National Guard members who were trying to overthrow the government. The war that ensued further destroyed the Nicaraguan society and economy, as did the embargo on Nicaraguan goods imposed by the United States in 1985. In 1987, after the United States stopped aid to the Contras, neither group could afford to continue the conflict, and peace was finally negotiated in 1991. Mrs. Violeta Chamarro was elected by popular vote as the first woman president of the continent, and in January 1997, Dr. Arnoldo Aleman Lacayo was elected, under the banner of a liberal alliance.

THE ANTHROPOLOGY OF MIGRATION

For Nicaragua, migration has been a way of life. Nicaragua has been permanently exposed to changes in its demographic characteristics because of the openness of its society and a multiplicity of historical factors. In Nicaragua, the major changes in cultural composition started after July 1979, when the end of the civil war brought to power the Sandinista regime. This was the period in history when the most massive migration took place. An estimated 700,000 Nicaraguans left their homeland at that time. For a population of merely 2 million people, this figure represented one-third of Nicaragua's citizens. Most people came to the United States, and fewer went to Costa Rica and other countries in the area (Organization of American States 1995).

The immediate factors that displaced Nicaraguans were fear and repression. Anyone who had been associated with the ousted regime had to flee or face brutality. Those Nicaraguans who did not leave were confronted with a major restructuring of the Nicaraguan society, mainly through the influence of the *internacionalistas,* a group of communists from all over the world who rapidly acquired major political and social prominence.

NICARAGUANS IN THE UNITED STATES

The quarter million Nicaraguans who came to live in the United States have shown a high morale and a great capacity to work hard. Overall, they have adapted well to the rules of the new, very complex American culture, proudly preserving the cultural and historical roots that link them to their homeland.

The first generations of Nicaraguans who were born in the United States are fully bilingual and have a high regard for education. In the city of Miami, Florida, where great concentrations of Nicaraguans live, issues of intercultural coexistence with the Cubans have been remarkable. The immediate cause for migration was very similar in the case of most Cubans and Nicaraguans. The geopolitical plans of international communism touched both countries at the heart of their nationalistic pride, but both groups have had an extraordinary ability not only to preserve their heritage in full but also to successfully adapt to life in the United States in a functional manner and create a successful community.

ISSUES OF CLINICAL RELEVANCE

Like other Hispanic groups in the United States, Nicaraguans come from a culture that adheres to traditional values, as described. Spanish is the predominant language of the immigrant generation, and Catholicism is the main religion. Family remains the most important institution of the group.

Nicaraguans, like other immigrant groups, have experienced residual psychological effects from the events that brought them to the United States and from the loss of their homeland. However, epidemiologic data indicate that although suicide and drug addiction have risen in the Nicaraguan society, they are less prevalent in the exile community, possibly confirming the principle of organic solidarity of migrant people when faced with hardship and challenge (Organization of American States 1995).

The most prevalent diagnoses among Nicaraguans in the United States are depression, anxiety, and posttraumatic stress disorder (PTSD). The following case vignettes have been selected to illustrate psychiatric issues that are pertinent to the Nicaraguan community.

The following case example illustrates low self-esteem in a woman who experienced previous abuse and a loss of professional status after immigrating to the United States and who had to become the head of the household.

Ms. H, a divorced woman in her 40s, sought psychiatric treatment because she was experiencing poor sleep, anxiety, weight loss, and tearfulness. She was the sole supporter of her two children but was employed in a low-paying position, even though she had had a professional career in Nicaragua. This greatly affected her self-esteem, and she was distressed that she could not do better. Her alcoholic ex-husband had verbally and physically abused her.

Treatment was started with an antidepressant, and weekly supportive therapy was successfully provided. The issues of low self-esteem in a woman who had come from a society of intricate *machismo* (the ideal of the strong, powerful, active man) and who had been abused were addressed in brief, focused psychotherapy. Eventually, Ms. H was able to obtain a better job, and she started dating a man who treated her with dignity and appreciation. At the monthly follow-up, her condition remained improved.

This case illustrates several issues that are relevant in working with Nicaraguan patients. First, this patient experienced a loss of professional status in immigrating to the United States. This has been the situation for many people who were professionals in their countries but in the United States are underemployed, not only in low-paying jobs but also in positions in which they are not able to use their skills. It is not atypical to see a former teacher cleaning houses or a former doctor working as a janitor in a hospital.

Second, this patient was the head of a household and was previously in an abusive relationship. Again, the experience of immigration has forced women to take on responsibilities they might not have had to assume in their homeland, such as working outside the home and being the primary breadwinner. However, it also has allowed them the opportunity to change circumstances that they might have been expected to tolerate in a more traditional setting, with a lingering abusive relationship.

The following case examples illustrate the importance of having a through understanding of patients' life circumstances in a patient with paranoia, a social marker of distress, and a patient with PTSD.

Mr. I, a college graduate in his 30s, went to Nicaragua to visit some friends and to reclaim some property that had been confiscated. While in Nicaragua, he developed intense fear, hid in his room, and refused to leave it. He began to think that the authorities were after him and that arrest warrants had been issued. When he returned to the United States, the intense paranoid delusion remained, along with elements of dysphoria and agitation. A brief psychotic disorder was diagnosed. He was treated with antipsychotic medications and weekly supportive psychotherapy. He responded successfully to treatment, and the medication was tapered. A year later, he remained symptom free.

Mr. J, a Nicaraguan man in his 40s, developed severe insomnia, flashbacks, and extreme apprehension several months after he arrived in the United States. His history revealed that while in Nicaragua, he had been imprisoned and subjected to subhuman, crowded conditions while incarcerated. He also developed intrusive, obsessional thinking and symptomatology of depression. He was given a diagnosis of PTSD. After brief psychotherapeutic intervention and temporary treatment with a sedative-hypnotic, Mr. J's symptoms remitted, and he was able to resume his normal life as a bank clerk.

In the above case examples, an understanding of Nicaragua's past and current political situation helped the clinician to understand the etiology of the symptoms and to commence the appropriate treatment. Traumatic experiences are often at the core of refugees' and immigrants' experiences, but they often remain undisclosed because of either the patient's inability to spontaneously bring them up or the clinician's reluctance to ask. People who have been tortured may feel shame, guilt, and helplessness or that it is useless to talk about their experiences because others simply will not understand. Similarly, therapists may inadvertently avoid opening up the discussion because of the difficulty in listening to stories of purposeful, horrifying brutality (Carrillo 1991; Lopez et al. 1988).

The following case example of a man with Alzheimer's disease illustrates several values that are important in Nicaraguan families and how these are affected by immigration.

Mr. L, an 85-year-old man, was brought to the doctor's office by his daughter because his memory was declining, he was wandering during the night, and he was making persistent claims that he was living on his farm in Nicaragua. After a thorough workup, he was given a diagnosis of advanced Alzheimer's disease. His daughter was very insistent on taking care of her father. She refused to place him in a nursing home because she was afraid "he would die there." She continued to take care of him, even though she lacked the financial resources, and eventually her stress became so prominent that she required antidepressant treatment.

The above case shows several values that are important in Nicaraguan families, including family loyalty and obligation and respect for and caregiving of the elderly. In Nicaragua, the daughter might have been able to help care for her father with the support of an extended family in a society accustomed to taking care of the elderly at home. But in the United States, her energy was focused on everyday survival, and being a caregiver of her father felt like another burden. Furthermore, the worsening of the father's condition may have been exacerbated by his own displacement (i.e., not knowing the language in the United States and lacking the familiarity of his homeland, neighborhood, and acquaintances to help orient him).

The following case illustrates some of the intergenerational conflicts that occur between immigrant parents and their children because they undergo different rates of acculturation (Bernal and Flores-Ortiz 1982).

> John, a 16-year-old boy, was brought to treatment by his mother, who was concerned about her son's "habits." She reported that he was reclusive and spent long hours in his room listening to heavy metal music and not participating in family life. She also reported that he wore torn and loose pants. The mother had been born and raised in Nicaragua, was Catholic, and did not agree with all these "fads," as she expressed it. On interview, it was clear that John was experiencing a mild depression. He had also begun to smoke marijuana but quit after experiencing two panic attacks. After several weeks of treatment with an antidepressant and psychotherapy, his depressive symptoms remitted, he completely quit smoking marijuana, and his relationship with his parents improved. John reported that even his mother had made changes, becoming more tolerant of his musical choices. He was euthymic at 1-year follow-up.

Parents often feel as if their authority is weakened when their children do not defer to them in a way that is culturally expected, and, similarly, children may feel that their parents' expectations are too restrictive. The therapist must become a communication broker between the parent and the child and must help them see the world through each other's lenses. Also, as in the above case, it is important not to overlook substance use as self-medication for depression.

REFERENCES

Bernal G, Flores-Ortiz Y: Latino families in therapy: engagement and evaluation. J Marital Fam Ther 8:357–365, 1982

Bethell L: Central America Since Independence. Cambridge, MA, Cambridge University Press, 1993

Carrillo E. Engaging the immigrant or refugee patient in treatment, in Immigrants and Refugees: A Handbook of Clinical Care. Edited by Lopez AG, Lee E, Farr F. San Francisco, CA, University of California San Francisco School of Medicine, 1991

Cuadra PA: El Nicaraguense. Managua, Nicaragua, Hispamericano, 1994

Lainez F: Nicaragua y sus Dilemas Historicos. Managua, Nicaragua, Cuadernos Anagrama, 1992

Lopez A, Boccellari A, Hall K: Posttraumatic stress disorder in a Central American refugee. Hospital and Community Psychiatry 39:1309–1311, 1988

Organization of American States: Statistical Summary. Washington, DC, Executive Secretariat of the Inter-American Drug Abuse Council, 1995

CHAPTER 10

Peruvians

Renato D. Alarcón, M.D., M.P.H.

PERU IS THE THIRD largest country in South America after Brazil and Argentina and the fourth most populated behind Colombia. It is generally accepted that its name originates from a Quechua word meaning "land of abundance." Pre-Colombian cultures of extraordinary accomplishments set the stage for the establishment of the Inca Empire, which around the tenth and eleventh centuries dominated about two-thirds of the territory that is South America today. The 1500s witnessed the collision of the European and the native cultures and the beginning of Peru's struggle with a *mestizo* (Spanish and American Indian) identity. During the Spanish colonial domination, Lima, the capital of the viceroyalty of Peru, was the most important political and economic center of the Americas. The independence wars led to the creation of the republic in the 1820s. Peru's current political organization is based on a representative democracy, with a president elected for 5-year terms and a unicameral congress. The country is divided into 24 departments with intendants appointed by the president. Although a violent guerrilla war conducted by two Maoist and Marxist groups has diminished considerably, the country still faces difficult times on both the political and the economic fronts (Alarcón 1995).

GEOGRAPHICAL CHARACTERISTICS

Peru is located in west central South America, bounded on the west by the Pacific Ocean, on the east by Brazil and Bolivia, on the north by Ecuador and

Colombia, and on the south by Chile. Peru's land can be divided into three main geographic regions: the coastal plain, the highlands or sierra, and the jungle or forest region. Some geographers would add the inter-Andean valleys and would divide the sierra region into temperate, high barren, and high Andes subregions.

The area of Peru is about 496,225 square miles, equivalent to the combined areas of Great Britain, France, and Spain. The land area is supplemented by 238,417 square miles of territorial waters reaching 200 miles into the Pacific Ocean. Peru is supported by three water systems: the Amazon River in the jungle, Lake Titicaca (the highest navigational lake on earth), and the Pacific Ocean.

DEMOGRAPHIC PATTERNS

Under the Incas, Peru's population reached 12 million, but during the first 50 years of Spanish rule, nearly 10 million Indians perished. From the time of the first census in 1793 to the mid-twentieth century, the population increased tenfold. The average annual population growth was 2% in the 1990s. The estimated 2000 population of Peru was 27,012,899, with an overall population density of about 17 people per square kilometer. The population structure is pyramidal; about 35% of the population is younger than 15 years, and 4% is 60 years or older.

About 52.6% of the population lives in the coastal plain (33% in Lima), but only 33.6% and 34.6% live in the highlands and the jungle, respectively. The sex distribution is about even: 50.4% male and 49.6% female. There is a trend toward urbanization, with 69.3% of the population in 1989 living in cities with more than 50,000 inhabitants and 30.7% living in rural areas. A social phenomenon similar to that seen in other Latin American countries is the high rate of urban decay and the significant growth of shantytowns at the periphery of major cities (Silva-Santisteban 1995).

ETHNIC AND CULTURAL CHARACTERISTICS

By the early 1990s, 47% of the population was of Quechua origin, 32% *mestizo*, 12% white, 5% Aymara, and 3% other groups, including blacks and Asians brought in as farm workers in the second half of the nineteenth century.

More than 92.5% of the Peruvians are practicing or nominal Roman Catholics, the official religion of Peru since 1915. About 5.5% are Protestants, with the number of churches of different denominations growing at a relatively rapid pace, particularly in the *barriadas* (shantytowns). Other religious groups include small numbers of Jews and Moslems.

Seventy percent of the people speak Spanish. In 1975, a leftist military government established Quechua, the language of the Inca Empire, as a second language, but the experiment failed. Aymara, spoken primarily by groups around Lake Titicaca in the southeastern part of the country bordering Bolivia, appears to be fading. Small and isolated tribal groups in the jungle speak other native dialects.

Peru's cultural history stems from the rich pre-Inca and Inca heritage and the many Spanish and European contributions. Archeological excavations have uncovered monumental pre-Inca and Inca remains, and the arts of the Spanish colonial period mixed with the native created extraordinary paintings, public and private buildings, churches, and music. Maintaining the Quechua and Aymara folklore and stimulating other cultural manifestations of the whites, *mestizos,* and blacks contributes to the cultural diversity that makes Peru one of the richest and most appealing countries in that regard. Even though the country's archeological riches have been dilapidated, many Peruvian museums in Lima and other important cities still show part of the proud accomplishments of the original Peruvians. Lima's National Library, founded in 1821, houses more than 3.2 million books (Pacheco-Velez 1988).

SOCIOECONOMIC REALITIES

Agriculture, forestry, fishing, and mining are the main economic activities in Peru. In the early 1990s, 34% of the total population was economically active, with 56% being older than 15. Female workers composed 38% of the workforce, and the unemployment rate of the country was 9%. The average household size was 5.2, with a mean income of less than $2,000 per year.

Inflation reached a high of 76.5% in 1990, but since then, several stabilization measures have proven successful. Trade has experienced an upward turn, even though the level of employment has not increased significantly. Privatization has been imposed in several key industries and economic sectors. Economic investment that seemed to be on the verge of significant growth has experienced a slowdown in the wake of recent political events in the Peruvian capital. Despite these difficulties, a sense of hope prevails among most of the Peruvian population at present.

Socioeconomic stratification is clear in Peru—only 4% of the families in 1996 received about 27% of the per capita income, whereas 18% had another 31% of the income. At the lower income levels, almost 80% of the population had only 42% of the national income. According to the 1991 Standard of Living Survey, 22% of the total population was living in extreme poverty, and 54% was in a state of critical poverty (Britannica Book of the Year 1996).

EDUCATION AND HEALTH

Public basic education in Peru is free and compulsory for all children between ages 6 and 15 years. In the late 1980s, 3.7 million pupils attended elementary schools, and about 1.7 million students were enrolled in secondary and vocational schools. Nevertheless, it is estimated that 20% of the population in Peru has no formal schooling. Thirty-three percent have less than a primary education, and only 5% enjoy higher education. The adult literate population rose from 42% in 1940 to about 85% in the mid-1980s. In 1994, the illiteracy rate in the population 15 years and older was 12%, with rates as high as 30% or more in some parts of the sierra region (Pan American Health Organization 1994).

Peru has 45 institutions of higher education and 16 schools of medicine, from which about 1,000 new physicians graduate each year. Twenty-one percent are women, but it is estimated that by 2010, at least one-third of the medical professionals will be women. The medical school career lasts 8 years; postgraduate training follows closely the American model of 3–4 years for generalists plus an additional 3–4 years for medical and surgical specialties.

Currently, there are about 25,000 physicians in the country, 1.13 for each 1,000 inhabitants. In 1990, there were 5,600 dentists, 18,000 nurses, 6,000 pharmacists, and 3,500 midwives. As in many other Latin American countries, up to 70% of the health professionals reside in the nation's capital.

A total of 400 hospitals were equally distributed between the government and private sectors (about 15 hospital beds per 10,000 people). Public health expenditures accounted for about 5.5% of the national budget, with only $17 per capita in public health expenditures and 0.28% devoted to mental health.

By the early 1990s, Peru had a mortality rate of 7.4 per 1,000, a birthrate of 29 per 1,000, and an infant mortality rate of 66.1 per 1,000 live births. In 2000, the infant mortality rate was 41 deaths per 1,000 live births. The average life expectancy in Peru is 72.5 years for women and 67.6 years for men. A cholera epidemic in 1991 killed more than 1,000 Peruvians and sickened another 150,000 (Mariateguí 1988; Pan American Health Organization 1994).

PERUVIANS IN THE UNITED STATES

The migratory patterns of Peruvians toward the United States do not resemble those of Mexico, Central America, or other countries in the northern part of South America. Peru is too distant for significant waves of immigration to the United States. Nevertheless, the trend of immigration to the United States seems to be growing, particularly among young people who want to further their education and training or, eventually, to stay. Also, the massive domination of American popular culture through technological means has no exception in Peru. Economic changes favoring imports and opening the markets have contributed to the growing influence of the United States and things American on the lives of Peruvians. The advent of American and transnational corporations creates imbalance, in the opinion of social scientists. As a result, cultural identity may diminish as much as the domestic industry's growth.

The ambivalent relationship between Latin American countries and the United States also is found among Peruvians. Political upheavals, although not infrequent, have not caused migratory waves. Peruvian immigrants are mostly from middle and lower middle social classes; these blue-collar workers go to the industrial states in the Northeast, in the Midwest, and on the West Coast. Yet, increasing numbers are coming to Florida, to the Southeast, to the Southwest, and even to some of the inland states in the Plains. An estimated 38,000 Peruvians have become American citizens in the last 25 years, whereas a total of more than 103,000 non–United States citizens entered the country during the same period. Currently, most of the Peruvian immigrants are located in the Northeast (50% total), with New York, New Jersey, and Connecticut leading the other states. Almost 4,900 United States citizens and 16,700 non–United States citizens live in Florida, and 11,300 United States citizens and 30,400 non–United States citizens live on the West Coast, mostly in California.

The number of Peruvian families entering the United States has diminished significantly since 1984; before that year, about 1,000 new families of naturalized Peruvians entered the country compared with an average of 200 since 1985. However, the number of families of noncitizens has been increasing steadily at a rate of 4,000–4,200 per year, raising the possibility that numerous Peruvians remain in this country with tourist visas or as illegal aliens. Also, more women than men from Peru seem to be entering the United States (U.S. Bureau of the Census 1996).

Because of factors such as distance, economic obstacles, and perhaps the fear of not being allowed back into the United States, few Peruvians engage in so-called back-and-forth migration. The acculturation and adaptation processes of these immigrants to the United States follow very much the pattern of other Latin Americans. As members of the working class, they congregate in areas of large cities where they can protect and maintain their level of cultural identity and intrafamily and interfamily relationships and enjoy restaurants, clubs, sports activities, religious festivities, and other community events. Particularly important is the well-entrenched devotion to the Lord of Miracles religious image, St. Rose of Lima, and St. Martin of Porras, the latter a mulatto Dominican monk who lived in the sixteenth century in

Lima and was made a saint by the pope in the 1950s.

Similarly, the fate of Peruvian professionals in the United States does not differ significantly from that of other Latin Americans. They also settle in localities near the big cities of the Northeast, West, or Midwest. Occasionally, some move to rural areas. For the most part, however, workers remain in metropolitan areas as employees of big factories, and their wives stay at home to care for their children or work part-time as domestic laborers.

Being a minority within a minority, Peruvians do not seem to play an active role in "ethnic politics." The differences between South Americans, Central Americans, Mexicans, Cubans, and Puerto Ricans have been highlighted on numerous occasions. There is not, of course, any indication of "national personalities," even though some cultural characteristics of everyday life may differ. Nevertheless, commonalities such as language and religion play a significant role in the relatively smooth integration of Peruvians with the larger Latin American and Hispanic communities in the United States.

MENTAL HEALTH ISSUES

The socioeconomic factors of poverty, unemployment, underdevelopment, political violence, internal migration, and narcotic traffic and drug abuse in significant segments of the population, particularly younger persons, set the stage for serious family and community disruptions, with the sequelae of mental illness, crime, and social dislocation. By mid-1992, it was estimated that at least 300,000 persons were forced to leave their places of origin because of the state of quasi–civil war in the Andean region. No epidemiologic studies have specifically addressed the Peruvian immigrants to the United States. We present next some statistics related to epidemiologic data among the Peruvian population in Peru. The avatars of migration, acculturation, and adaptation to the host society of the United States may create some vulnerability in subgroups of Peruvian immigrants, according to well-accepted tenets of clinical epidemiology.

In a study of people living in a middle-class district of metropolitan Lima (Mariateguí and Adis-Castro 1970), 18.8% of those surveyed were given diagnoses of a psychiatric disorder. More than half of the sample were women; single persons had fewer mental disorders than was expected (widows and widowers were more affected), and less educated persons showed higher levels of psychiatric disturbance. Within the family constellation, mothers and wives showed higher percentages of disorders (32.4% and 27.4%, respectively). Unemployment and mental disorders were closely related. Likewise, 59% of those with a psychiatric diagnosis belonged to low socioeconomic groups.

Only 44.7% of the subgroup with psychiatric disorders consulted mental health professionals or folk healers.

In terms of diagnostic categories, neurosis, personality disorders, and child psychiatric disorders constituted two-thirds of the disorders compared with only 12% in the general population. Of the subgroup with psychiatric disorders, 29% had a diagnosis of neurosis, 18% had personality disorders, 16% had childhood disorders, 9% had alcoholism, 8% had convulsive disorders, 7% had mental retardation, 6% had psychosomatic conditions, and 6% had psychosis.

Of the neuroses, 3.2% were anxiety disorders, 1.3% were somatoform disorders, 1.0% were depressive disorders, and 0.1% were obsessive-compulsive disorder. Among the childhood disorders, anxiety disorders represented 1.8% of the general sample, conduct disorders represented 1.0%, and organic disorders represented 0.2%. Of the psychoses, schizophrenia represented 0.5% of the general sample, bipolar disorders represented 0.7%, and psychotic depression represented 0.6%.

Alcoholism is a significant problem in the Peruvian population. In some of the poorest parts of metropolitan Lima, the rate has been up to 8.8%, with most alcoholic patients being migrants from Andean towns. In the same areas, 42.6% of a sample received psychiatric diagnoses. The internal migration has produced a condition known as *psychosomatic syndrome of maladaptation*, characterized by a variety of physical symptoms, demoralization, depression, and social disorganization.

Another epidemiologic study conducted in 1982 by the National Institute of Mental Health in a marginal district of Lima found a 41% prevalence of mental disorders. This rate is among the highest in Latin America. Particularly among the poorest and the youngest, the consumption of crack cocaine and cocaine is on the rise in the urban areas of Peru (Perales 1993).

In the early 1980s, mental disorders represented 2.03% of the diagnoses in those discharged from hospitals. This figure decreased to 1.65% in 1990 and was 1.83% in 1991. Young adults are at highest risk for a mental disorder or death as a result of acts of violence or accidents. In the Lima metropolitan area, more than 80% of all the complaints filed for assault involved women aged 20–39 years as victims.

Quality of life and life expectancy are significantly correlated. Despite its significance, mental health is not a priority in public health budgets or policies; in 1989, only 0.28% of the government's budget was devoted to mental health. Well-known psychosocial realities such as chronicity trends, unemployment, increasing rehabilitation costs, suicidal risks, lower life expectancy, increased violence and criminality, and lack of insurance or adequate social services create a potential for even more serious social problems.

A study of hospital epidemiology in Lima showed that the prevalence of substance abuse was massively predominant among males, with an age at onset that reached a peak between 22 and 24 years. Being single, attending secondary education, being unemployed, and having an age at onset between 9 and 19 years were the most salient variables. Crack cocaine, marijuana, tranquilizers, stimulants, barbiturates, narcotics, and inhalants were the drugs abused most often. Personality problems, schizophrenia, and alcohol abuse were the most frequent comorbid disorders.

The mental health system in Peru is mostly based on a significant public sector, moderate-sized Social Security and private sectors, and a very small academic sector. The public sector is generally weak and mostly oriented toward the care of chronically ill patients; it has minimal infrastructure and reduced personnel. Integration between different components of this sector is absent. Large state hospitals or even modern establishments such as the National Institute of Mental Health have a recurrent shortage of medications, equipment, linen, and other minimal requirements.

The Social Security sector has grown in recent years, its administration has improved, and a better organized network of satellite clinics and outreach programs promises better delivery of care. The financial crisis of the last decades has, however, militated against a systematic growth. The private sector is relatively small but certainly provides care that may be comparable to that of some facilities in developed countries. It is accessible to only the wealthy class in luxurious clinics located in exclusive sectors of the capital and other big cities and staffed primarily by foreign-trained physicians.

The academic sector is very small; teaching sites are mostly public or semiprivate establishments where trainees can learn to treat a variety of psychiatric conditions (see the next section, "Mental Health Training").

Psychopharmacology and psychotherapy are the preferred modalities of treatment. Most professionals use a combination of these therapeutic approaches. Psychoanalysis has significantly grown in Peru in the last three decades.

MENTAL HEALTH TRAINING

Peru has slightly over 1,200 psychiatrists, or about 1 per 1,918 persons. Psychologist numbers are about three times larger, but there are many fewer social workers and other mental health providers. Six psychiatric training programs exist, four of which are academically based. About 20–25 new psychiatrists graduate from these programs per year. The training is usually 3 years and follows the traditional rotations of inpatient, outpatient, consultation-liaison, addiction psychiatry, and electives. Most of the programs are multisite, a characteristic that, on the one hand, ensures diversity of exposure and clinical experience but, on the other hand, gives the trainees an uneven quality of teaching. The theoretical emphasis is eclectic, even though competing schools of phenomenological/biological and psychodynamic/psychoanalytical orientation are dominant. Among the mental health professionals, psychologists are the most progressive in psychoanalytical circles or in new and developing cognitive-behavioral approaches. No national examinations or certification tests are given at the end of the training period. Only a tiny minority of psychiatrists migrate to Europe or the United States to further their professional education, but more than two-thirds of those who migrate choose to stay abroad.

Critics of the current status of medical and psychiatric education in Latin American countries such as Peru emphasize the lack of integration between existing curricula and the sociocultural realities and actual mental health needs of the population. Research is not a priority in these programs, and the poverty of resources to sustain systematic efforts (both preclinical and clinical) makes for very limited accomplishments, with the exception of some countries and clinical areas such as epidemiology, sociocultural studies, and syndromic descriptions. Finally, the competition between psychiatrists and other mental health professionals and between mental health professionals and native healers may become an important component of the future evolution of mental health in Peru and the Latin American continent as a whole (Miguez 1995).

Multidisciplinary work appears to be developing consistently, particularly in urban areas. Psychologists are moving from the mere administration of psychometric tests to areas such as individual and group therapy, vocational assessment and rehabilitation, industrial and educational psychology, and cognitive-behavioral work. Social workers also are making inroads in case management, psychosocial diagnosis and assessment, information science, and counseling.

Community psychiatry and community mental health are developing with a mixture of academic interests, research projects, and actual delivery of services. The use of community leaders and organizations, as well as other professionals such as teachers, priests, police officers, and neighborhood organizations, is creating a climate favorable for the analysis and eventual alleviation of some social psychopathology.

MENTAL ILLNESS AND SOCIETY

As in many other countries, in Peru a great deal of social stigma is attached to mental illnesses. Even though the degree of tolerance to mental illness among families appears to be higher than in developed countries, issues such as shame, guilt, rejection, and social exclusion arise, particularly in marginal urban areas and metropolitan parts of the country. Mental illness is strongly attached to homelessness, perhaps at rates higher than 60%. Most of the Peruvian population is not sophisticated about the etiology and pathogenesis of mental illnesses. In addition, the tendency is to consider all mental illnesses as one, which certainly increases the levels of stigmatization and avoidance. Not infrequently, other professionals or nonpsychiatric medical practitioners contribute to the collective sense of rejection of mental illness as they unwittingly speak in a derisive way about such conditions and those who have them.

The most popular explanatory models of mental illness attribute it to either religious factors (punishment) or evil influences; sexual aberrations (such as masturbation); or disloyalty, treason, and deception. One of the most popular beliefs, however, is that mental illness is a sign of weakness, something that "macho" men do not experience and only "feminine" men or weaklings do experience.

In rural areas, Andean towns, and jungle villages, the belief in magic and its influence in causing mental conditions is rampant. Myths, fantasy, legend, and the transmission of a distorted oral history contribute to this phenomenon. Several culture-bound syndromes considered as variations of others known in different parts of the world are dominant. Significant among them are *susto* (fright illness), "heartbreak," "stolen soul," "possession," and related dissociative phenomena.

A gradual but sustained penetration of modern notions of mental illness has occurred, even in remote parts of the country. The growth of communication media and the easier access to those remote areas have contributed to this. Likewise, the use of medications (particularly major tranquilizers, anxiolytics, and antidepressants) is a noteworthy factor in the process. The figure of the doctor enjoys universal respect, admiration, and a sense of dependency that may contribute to acceptable degrees of medication compliance. However, this is not a generalized phenomenon, and poverty, inaccessibility of services, lack of professional attention, and chaotic administration of health programs make the follow-up and ultimately the prognosis of mental illnesses somber or, at best, uncertain (Alarcón 1990).

On the positive side, the strength of family, religious faith, and religious beliefs and a sense of deep solidarity among neighbors, acquaintances, and friends indicate a strong potential for social networks that can contribute to a wider degree of tolerance to and a better management of mental illnesses. This is particularly true in semirural and rural areas where mental patients are easily involved in everyday work in the fields, incipient commercial endeavors, little flea markets, and other community activities.

TREATMENT IN PERUVIAN PATIENTS

Peruvian patients, particularly those living in the United States, should be treated with a comprehensive approach to their double condition of carriers of a diagnosed mental disorder and foreigners in a different culture. In this context, some general characteristics relevant to their clinical management include the following:

- Strong notions of family and family unity, with a concomitant need to preserve its integrity at all costs, sometimes even at the risk of perpetuating dysfunctional group patterns, worsening of clinical conditions, or operation of rigid intrafamily rules
- Significant predominance of religious values both in the interpretive or explanatory models of illness and in the possibility of hope for success in treatment interventions (These values also expand to the creation or strengthening of social support networks.)
- Guardedness, a strong sense of privacy, shame related to potential stigma, and difficulty in "opening up" in therapeutic encounters, particularly at the beginning (In this context, patients prefer individual over group treatments.)
- Pride that both reinforces privacy and generates a degree of resilience toward negative experiences (It also reflects cultural issues such as *machismo*, courage in the face of adversity, persistent struggle, and refusal to accept defeat.)
- Proneness to idealism and idealization of events, figures, specific situations, dates, and so forth (These are linked with strong romanticism and a tendency toward abstract, theoretical thinking that may be useful in psychotherapeutic approaches.)
- Strong cultivation of friendship and determined efforts to preserve the feelings associated with it, such as loyalty, identification, and support (These feelings may result, at times, in the loss of some sense of realism in the light of interpersonal events.)
- Respect for authority and authority figures, including parents, law enforcement officers, priests, teachers, or doctors (Nevertheless, strong re-

pression may be used and, thus, at times emerge in the form of passive-aggressive behavior or open rebelliousness in interpersonal transactions.)

- Tendency to be easily disappointed, which translates into dramatic outbursts of emotional lability, anger, frustration, open regret, and tendency to catastrophize breakups in all kinds of relationships
- Tendency to overtly somatize as an "idiom of distress" in the face of adversity, depressogenic or anxiogenic events, and interpersonal difficulties (These also may appear as part of resistance to treatment, avoidance of responsibilities, or denial of symptoms or need for help.)
- Tendency to have explosive, irritable outbursts as disproportionate responses to different kinds of stimuli (These tendencies sometimes evolve into open irrationality, impulsiveness, and verbal or physical aggressiveness.)
- Open, sometimes theatrical or histrionic expressions of affection, admiration, and other positive emotions (These emotional states are loudly verbalized and expressed.)

REFERENCES

Alarcón RD: Identidad de la Psiquiatrìa Latinoamericana: Voces y Exploraciones en Torno a una Ciencia Solidaria. Mexico, Distrito Federal, Siglo XXI Editores, 1990

Alarcón RD: Perú, in Enciclopedia Iberoamericana de Psiquiatrìa, Vol 1. Edited by Vidal G, Alarcón RD, Lolas F. Buenos Aires, Argentina, Editorial Mèdica Panamericana, 1995, pp 519–520

Britannica Book of the Year: World Data. Chicago, IL, Encyclopedia Britannica, 1996

Lemlij M: Refexiones Sobre La Violencia. Lima, Peru, Society Anónima, 1994

Mariategui J: Salud Mental y Realidad Nacional: El Primer Quinqenio del Instituto Nacional de Salud Mental. Lima, Peru, Editorial Minerva, 1988

Mariateguí J, Adis-Castro G (eds): Estudios Sobre Epidemiología Psiquiátrica en Amèrica Latina. Buenos Aires, Argentina, Acta-Fondo para la Salud Mental, 1970

Miguez HA: Hombres y temas en la epidemiología de Amèrica Latina, in Enciclopedia Iberoamericana de Psiquiatrìa, Vol 2. Edited by Vidal G, Alarcón RD, Lolas F. Buenos Aires, Argentina, Editorial Mèdica Panamericana, 1995, pp 542–543

Pacheco-Velez C: Peru Promesa. Lima, Peru, Graficas emege de Forum, 1988

Pan American Health Organizations: Health Conditions in the Americas, Vol II (Scientific Publ No 549). Washington, DC, Pan American Health Organizations, 1994

Perales A: Salud mental en el Perú. Anales de Salud Mental 8:83–107, 1993

Silva-Santisteban F: Historia de Nuestro Tiempo: Testimonios. Lima, Peru, Editorial Universo, 1995

U.S. Bureau of the Census: Foreign-Born Population in the United States: Perú. Washington, DC, U.S. Bureau of the Census, 1996

CHAPTER 11

Puerto Ricans

Ian A. Canino, M.D.

Glorisa Canino Stolberg, Ph.D.

MIGRATION HISTORY

The migration of island Puerto Ricans to the mainland United States can be divided into three distinct periods (Stevens-Arroyo and Diaz-Stevens 1982). During the first period (1900–1945), most Puerto Ricans went to New York City. This period coincided with the arrival of contracted agricultural and industrial labor. Smaller groups of agricultural contract laborers also settled in less urban areas such as Hawaii, California, Arizona, and Ohio (Senior and Watkins 1966). During the second period (1946–1964), the largest numbers of Puerto Ricans arrived, increasing the New York City communities and expanding to other parts of New York; New Jersey; Connecticut; Chicago, Illinois; Pennsylvania; and the rest of the United States. In the 1940s, migrants were primarily urban, skilled, and predominantly women. In the 1950s, migrants were rural, unskilled, and predominantly male. The last period of migration started in 1965 and was termed the *revolving-door migration*. This period was characterized by a fluctuating pattern of net migration and a greater dispersion to other parts of the United States. Currently, many Puerto Ricans migrate to larger cities in the mainland United States from large cities in Puerto Rico, others migrate from small towns to small towns, and many others migrate in multiple diverse combinations.

Many explanations for this migration have been cited, including economic factors such as better job opportunities, overpopulation of the island, encouragement by the island government, the wish of stateside employers for cheap labor, and the low rates of air transportation (C. Rodriguez 1989). In contrast to other migrant groups, Puerto Ricans arrive as citizens, have accessible transportation to their country of origin, and serve in the United States armed forces (C. Rodriguez 1989).

DEMOGRAPHICS

The mainland Puerto Rican population currently constitutes the third largest United States Latino group. It accounts for 9.6% of the total Latino population of 31.7 million (Therrien and Ramirez 2000).Compared with the general United States population, Puerto Ricans are younger, have lower educational attainment, earn less, are more likely to be unemployed, and live below the poverty line. In comparison with other Latino groups, Puerto Ricans have the highest percentage of families below the poverty level (Therrien and Ramirez 2000), have younger mothers, and consequently have younger children in the household (Wasserman et al. 1994). In spite of this, a growing group has entered the middle class (Rivera-Batiz and Santiago 1995). Mainland Puerto Ricans tend to have higher mortality rates than do other Hispanics, but these rates are still lower than those of non-Hispanics (Rosenwaike 1987). Puerto Ricans have the highest prevalence of low-birthweight infants, and their children have the highest prevalence of chronic medical conditions when compared with Mexican Americans and Cuban Americans (Mendoza et al. 1991).

Mainland Puerto Ricans are a diverse group in terms of area of residence, unemployment rates, exposure to other ethnic groups, and level of acculturation. Although still concentrated in the Northeast, they have established communities in the Midwest, Texas, and increasingly in the Southeast, mainly in Florida. Because of their large migration after World War II, Puerto Ricans now include several generations, from those with many decades of residency in the United States to those newly arrived. Many Puerto Ricans have lived for extended periods on both the island of Puerto Rico and the mainland United States.

Between 1980 and 1990, the labor force participation of Puerto Rican women increased, and the occupational distribution of all Puerto Ricans on the mainland was significantly upgraded. This did not offset the overall high unemployment rate during the same period, perhaps because of the decrease in labor participation of the men and the shift of employment from manufacturing to other sectors of the economy (Rivera-Batiz and Santiago 1995).

In an analysis of 1990 census data for 49 metropolitan areas with 40,000 or more Puerto Ricans, a considerable variation in the level of segregation between them, blacks, and whites was found in terms of regional location, size of the metropolitan area, and total size of the Puerto Rican population. High levels of segregation were associated with the older Puerto Rican communities, decentralization of unemployment, and low levels of suburbanization (Santiago 1992).

In terms of acculturation, an intergenerational study of Puerto Rican families in New York (Rogler and Cooney 1984) found that the greatest changes occurred in socioeconomic status, values and self-concept, language used at home, and bicultural preferences. As education in the next generation increased, so did the knowledge of English and Spanish, even though the use of Spanish decreased. The subjects with more education were less fatalistic, less family oriented, and more modern. Age at arrival had an important effect on ethnic self-identification and was related to language ability and usage. Those who arrived at a younger age reported more frequent use of English.

These generational, geographical, and acculturation patterns are particularly relevant because increases in levels of acculturation have been associated with an increase in the use of health services (Vega et al. 1999). In a recent study, first-generation Puerto Ricans reported that they were less healthy in general when compared with their second-generation counterparts (Cortez and Rogler 1996).

RESEARCH AND CLINICAL FINDINGS

Research Findings

> Now it is clear that to be culturally valid, comparative epidemiological and clinical studies need to do more than to follow a rigorous model of translation, back-translation, semantic adjustment, and validation of instruments. Cross-cultural validity can occur only when indigenous categories of experience are incorporated into assessment schedules. Otherwise, research will remain a kind of colonial imposition of Western categories on experiences, some of which are shared but many of which differ in important ways. (Guarnaccia et al. 1990, p. 1455)

Many studies of Latinos do not differentiate among the different groups, others are unable to oversample for specific subgroups, and many do not study intragroup differences. It is difficult to assess, for example, whether the mental health profiles of third-generation Puerto Ricans are closer to their third-generation Mexican American counterparts or to their non–Puerto Rican neighbors. It is often assumed that first generations of migrants express cultural patterns of behavior more similar to their country of origin than to their host country.

Despite brave attempts among some researchers to address the above-mentioned methodological concerns, additional fiscal and political obstacles have hindered the study of large numbers of mainland Puerto Ricans in terms of their mental health. In view of these limitations, in this section, we address some, but not all, of the studies that have been done in specific areas relevant to, but not exclusively in or representative of, all mainland Puerto Ricans. A review of studies of island Puerto Ricans is inevitable and perhaps applicable to a subgroup of mainland Puerto Ricans with low acculturation levels.

Depression

When mainland Puerto Ricans are compared with the general population and with Cuban and Mexican Americans, they have higher rates of depressive symptomatology even after controlling for socioeconomic differences (Moscicki et al. 1989). However, when compared with low-income island Puerto Ricans, as measured by the Center for Epidemiologic Studies Depression Scale (CES-D), mainland Puerto Ricans have similar rates. Low educational level, gender, low household income, and unemployment were predictors in both samples (Vera et al. 1991). Guarnaccia et al. (1990) discussed these findings by questioning the validity of the nosological system in which the instruments are used and explaining the potential influence of the fact that Puerto Ricans are exposed to more social stressors than are either Mexican Americans or Cuban Americans in the United States. Canino (1994) explained that these findings may be caused by the added stressors of migration, the disruption of social and family systems, and the prejudice experienced by this group. She added, though, that the limitations of the cultural sensitivity of the instruments used and the lack of concurrent ethnographic research must be considered before any final conclusions are made.

Conversely, for both mainland and island Puerto Ricans, depressive disorders were more than twice as prevalent in women as in men (10.7% vs. 4.9%), and the prevalence of dysthymia was almost four times greater in women than in men (G. Canino et al. 1987b; Moscicki et al. 1989). In the Puerto Rico study, even after demographics and health, marital, and employment status variables were controlled for in multiple regression analyses, women continued to be at higher risk for depressive symptomatology than men were. Consistent with other studies, separated, widowed, or divorced individuals; those with poor physical or mental health; unemployed males; and those residing in urban areas had more depressive symptoms than their counterparts. The difference in the prevalence of depressive disorders between males and females was more marked among island Puerto Ricans than among the U.S. population of the Epidemiologic Catchment Area (ECA) study, in whom the sex differences were not as dramatic. The higher sex ratio in Puerto Rico than in the United States is consistent with a gender role model that postulates that Latino males and females have different vulnerability to depressive disorders because of the more patriarchal social context in which they are socialized.

Illicit Drug Use and Abuse

Latinos in general seem to report lower rates of illicit drug use and abuse. Considerably lower prevalence rates of illicit drug use (8.2%) and drug abuse and dependence syndromes (1.2%) were found in Puerto Rico than in five United States communities reported by the ECA surveys (average of 30.4% and 8.8%, respectively) (Anthony and Helzer 1991; G. Canino et al. 1993).

The difference in prevalence rates of drug use and abuse between sites could not be explained by differences in the age distributions across the two survey populations. Because the island sample was younger (it included no persons older than 69) and because illicit drug use is more common among 18- to 39-year-olds than among older adults, the island prevalence might have been expected to be higher, not lower. The lower rates of drug use and abuse in Puerto Rico were consistent with findings obtained from other Latino populations in both the United States and South America. For example, the prevalence of drug abuse and dependence among the Mexican American immigrants at the Los Angeles, California, ECA site was 1.8% (Anthony and Helzer 1991). The rates of drug addiction were much higher for Mexican Americans born in the United States, suggesting that acculturation to the United States society may be related to higher rates of drug use. These findings were replicated by Vega et al. (1998) in a study of Mexican Americans from Fresno, California. Similarly, rates of marijuana use were higher for Mexicans living in the United States (42%) than for Mexicans living in Mexico (7%) (Ortiz and Medina-Mora 1988). Although the possibility that Latinos generally tend to underreport drug use compared with whites or acculturated Latinos cannot be ruled out, cultural differences between these populations might explain the findings obtained. It would seem worthwhile to consider in future research whether the apparent differences might be due to greater familism and extended kinship networks existent in Latino and Puerto Rican families in particular. The higher rates of family conflict, disintegration, and alienation sometimes found in the families of those with drug abuse and dependence are less common in Puerto Rico, especially compared with white and Latino populations in the bigger cities of the United States.

Alcohol Abuse and Dependence

A comparison of the epidemiology of alcohol abuse and dependence in the Diagnostic Interview Schedule (DIS)–based population surveys carried out in 10 different regions of the world showed considerable variation in the prevalence of the disorder across sites (Helzer and Canino 1992). However, in those regions where Latinos were studied, it became apparent that alcoholism was the most frequent disorder in the populations of island Puerto Ricans and Mexican Americans (G. Canino et al. 1992). Although the symptom expressions and course of alcoholism were similar across several cultures, age at onset and sex differences were observed. For most of the sites, the mean age at onset of first symptoms was in the early to mid-20s. A later mean age at onset (late 20s and early 30s) was found in Puerto Rico and among Mexican Americans of Los Angeles. The later age at onset in Puerto Ricans and Mexican Americans was interpreted as the result of the greater tolerance of these Latino groups for intoxication and alcoholic behavior among men. It was hypothesized that symptomatic alcoholic behavior may not be endorsed until it is more severely expressed (G. Canino et al. 1992).

Although in all the cultures studied, excessive drinking and alcoholism were predominantly male activities, the male-to-female ratio varied considerably across cultures. The sex ratios were particularly high in the Asian and Latino cultures (where alcoholism was considerably more common in men) as compared with the Western and Anglo-Saxon cultures. In the communities studied, alcoholism was 4–6 times greater in men than in women. In Seoul, Korea; Puerto Rico; and the United States Mexican American populations, alcoholism was between 12 and 25 times greater in men. The differences in sex ratios across cultures provided evidence in favor of the importance of culture and attitudes toward drinking in determining the prevalence rates. In the more traditional cultures with marked gender role stereotypes (as in Puerto Rico and among Mexican Americans), the prevalence of excessive drinking and alcoholism among women was considerably lower than in the less traditional cultures. Of interest, nevertheless, was that among the young age groups of Puerto Ricans (17–25 years), the sex ratio in the prevalence of alcoholism was considerably diminished to that observed in the United States, suggesting that with new and future generations, the prevalence of alcoholism in women would be increasingly higher than at present (G. Canino et al. 1987a).

As with drug addiction, the rate of alcoholism increased among Mexican Americans proportionately with the number of years living in the United States, suggesting that higher acculturation to the United States society or the stress associated with the migration experience and the discrimination experienced by this minority group could be associated with a higher risk for alcoholism (G. Canino et al. 1992). Both of these findings may apply to mainland Puerto Ricans with similar experiences, but large research studies are still lacking.

Somatization Disorder

Somatization disorder and somatic symptoms seem to be more prevalent among Latino populations than among other ethnic groups. Clinical studies have reported that Latino patients interviewed both in the United States and in their countries of origin tend to have higher levels of somatic symptoms than do their non-Latino counterparts (Escobar et al. 1983; Mezzich and Raab 1980). Because even in more developed countries people of lower socioeconomic backgrounds who have a psychiatric disorder are more likely than those of more advantaged backgrounds to have somatic symptoms, the tendency to "somatize" rather than "psychologize" has been viewed as being largely the result of socioeconomic factors.

This association with sociodemographic factors was confirmed in a psychiatric epidemiology study carried out in the island of Puerto Rico (I. Canino et al. 1992; Rubio-Stipec et al. 1993). However, the higher mean number of somatic symptoms in Puerto Ricans as compared with other groups (ECA communities, Mexican Americans, and non-Hispanic whites) could not be solely explained by differences in age, sex, level of education, and number of people in the household. This difference remained significant after statistically taking into account sample differences in age, sex, and education (I. Canino et al. 1992).

Previous explorations of those findings determined that this tendency of Puerto Ricans to somatize was not related to what has been commonly stated as a tendency to express depressive symptoms or demoralization through somatic symptoms (Rubio-Stipec et al. 1989). In this study, Rubio-Stipec and others used symptom data from the 1984 adult probability sample of residents in Puerto Rico and found that five clusters of items (those associated with diagnoses of affective disorders, schizophrenia, phobic disorder, somatization, and alcoholism) were formed. The factor structure of these scales was replicated in two probability samples of the Los Angeles ECA study, one composed of Mexican Americans and one of Anglo-Americans. Four of the scales were replicated in both Los Angeles samples, but the scale of somatization was not formed in either of the Los Angeles samples, only in the Puerto Rico sample. Of interest, however, was that the depressive and somatization scales formed through the factor analyses were separate and did not contain overlapping items, suggesting that both depressive and somatization symptoms are separate and distinct constructs.

Another possible explanation for this high prevalence of somatic symptoms was explored. In the probing system of the DIS used to separate physically explained from possible, the respondent reports a symptom, then he or she is asked whether a doctor was told about it and if so what the doctor said was causing the symptom. If the doctor said that the symptom was explained by a physical illness, it is not counted toward the diagnosis or as a somatic symptom. If Puerto Rican doctors are more prone to interpret somatic symptoms as "psychogenic," then this could explain the higher prevalence of the symptoms.

Another possible explanation is related to the accessibility of health care. In countries where health care is not as accessible (for whatever reason) or people do not seek health care as readily, many people with physical symptoms might not see a physician, and if no cause is attributed by the respondent, physical symptoms might be classified as symptoms of somatization disorder. For this reason, the probe chart of somatization was examined by the Composite International Diagnostic Interview (CIDI), which is the same used by the DIS, to ascertain its effectiveness in truly classifying somatic symptoms as psychiatric symptoms (Rubio-Stipec et al. 1993). Data generated from 16 countries (many of which are underdeveloped and have poor accessibility of care) in the first field trial of the CIDI were used to test the interrater reliability of each coding and to examine whether the sum of symptoms classified under the probe flowchart was associated with the known correlates of somatization. The findings showed that the probe flowchart screens somatic symptoms similarly in a variety of settings and cultures and that it is highly reliable for each of its five possible coding classifications. Therefore, comparisons of the rates of somatic symptoms between different sites and cultures with the somatization module helped identify true cultural differences. In fact, the findings showed a higher prevalence of somatic symptoms among populations of all Latin countries as compared with those of other cultural heritages. This is consistent with the results of previous clinical and epidemiologic studies quoted above.

To explain cultural differences in the presentation of somatic and psychological symptoms, it has been argued that some groups (e.g., Anglo-Saxons) may be more likely to partition somatic and psychological phenomena in a Cartesian way (mind-body dichotomy), whereas others (e.g., Latin Americans) may be more likely to integrate both kinds of experiences and express them somatically. Our study of this issue suggested that for Puerto Ricans and other Latin populations, this theory might be true.

Clinical Findings

> People use their cultural knowledge and skills differently in varied settings. Different social settings demand different interaction styles, language uses, and deployment of knowledge. When illness or other problems occur, people may emphasize their native culture as a source of comfort or support, or may emphasize the host's culture approaches both to distant themselves from the pain of illness and to mobilize resources available in the new setting. (Guarnaccia and Rodriguez 1996, p. 431)

Clinical issues relevant to mainland Puerto Ricans have to be understood within the context that many cultural norms are frequently being revised, are adjusting to new demands, and are being influenced by other cultural groups in the vicinity. Cultural values and beliefs are often affected by life experiences and may be adaptive or nonadaptive. The effect of stress, social class, and physical or psychiatric disorders on cultural norms needs to be considered as well. Guarnaccia and Rodriguez (1996) advised clinicians to be careful in focusing on generalized values and concepts of illness that can lead to stereotyping. In the following review, we address those values that are thought to be the most relevant.

Language/Idioms of Distress

The acquisition of a second language often enriches the native language, and bilingualism is associated with higher levels of cognitive attainment (Hakuta and Garcia 1989). Education, regional differences, and socioeconomic status also influence language. In recently migrated Spanish-speaking Puerto Ricans, the rate of language acquisition, as well as the context and frequency of language use, may vary. They may speak English at the workplace and in school, but not at home, or may use both languages interchangeably in all or some settings. Second- or third-generation Puerto Ricans may act as language brokers to their compatriots who arrived more recently and may acquire additional skills as translators or interpreters. Unfortunately, many eventually become English dominant or monolingual in English.

There has been an increased interest in the literature about culture-specific idioms, words, and expressions that are used to communicate distress and, at times, symptoms. Clinicians must be aware of the meaning and the nuances of these expressions so that they can understand and interpret what the patient really means. In addition, in a study assessing whether idioms of distress have mental health significance, Rogler and colleagues (1994) found that idioms of distress based on anger and injustice were correlated widely with professionally developed measures of anxiety, depression, and somatization (anger) and with the use of professional mental health care (perceived injustice).

Those idioms of distress that have been described that are thought to be relevant to Puerto Ricans are *nervios, ataques de nervios, locura,* and *celajes. Nervios* has been defined as "a vulnerability of experiencing symptoms of depression, anxiety, dissociation, somatization and rarely psychosis or poor impulse control given interpersonal frustrations" (Lewis-Fernandez 1996, p. 159) or

> a general state of vulnerability to stressful life experiences and to a syndrome brought on by difficult life circumstances. The term *nervios* includes a wide range of symptoms of emotional distress, somatic disturbance, and inability to function. Common symptoms include headaches and 'brain aches,' irritability, stomach disturbances, sleep difficulties, nervousness, easy tearfulness, inability to concentrate, trembling, tingling sensations, and *mareos* (dizziness with occasional vertigolike exacerbations)....*Nervios* is a very broad syndrome that spans the range from cases free of a mental disorder to presentations resembling Adjustment, Anxiety, Depressive, Dissociative, Somatoform, or Psychotic Disorders. (American Psychiatric Association 2000, p. 901)

Ataques de nervios are "acute, fit-like exacerbations of *nervios"* (Guarnaccia et al. 1989; Lewis-Fernandez 1996).

> Commonly reported symptoms include uncontrollable shouting, attacks of crying, trembling, heat in the chest rising into the head, and verbal or physical aggression. Dissociative experiences, seizurelike or fainting episodes, and suicidal gestures are prominent in some attacks but absent in others. A general feature of an *ataque de nervios* is a sense of being out of control. *Ataques de nervios* frequently occur as a direct result of a stressful event relating to the family....*Ataques* span the range from normal expressions of distress not associated with having a mental disorder to symptom presentations associated with the diagnosis of Anxiety, Mood, Dissociative, or Somatoform Disorders. (American Psychiatric Association 2000, p. 899)

A scale to measure this popular category of distress was developed by Guarnaccia and colleagues (1989). Approximately 23% of the adult population of Puerto Rico fit the *"ataques de nervios"* category described in the scale. Also, women, those of low socioeconomic status, formerly married persons, and those out of the labor force were significantly overrepresented in the *ataques* group. In addition, a significant proportion of those scoring high on the scale met diagnostic criteria for a DSM-III (American Psychiatric Association 1980) disorder. Particularly high rates of major depression, dysthymia, agoraphobia, phobic disorder, and panic disorder were found among the *ataque de nervios* group.

Locura is

> A term used by Latinos in the United States and Latin America to refer to a severe form of chronic psychosis. The condition is attributed to an inherent vulnerability, to the effect of multiple life difficulties, or to a combination of both factors. Symptoms exhibited by persons with locura include incoherence, agitation, auditory and visual hallucinations, inability to follow rules of social interaction, unpredictability, and possible violence. (American Psychiatric Association 2000, p. 901)

Swerdlow (1992) found in a small study of Puerto Ricans who had schizophrenia and who were living in New York that their belief and their community's belief that their illness was not *locura* but *nervios* helped. According to the author, this minimized social stigmatization and facilitated continued social involvement.

Finally, *celajes* is a word frequently used by Puerto Ricans that means "seeing shadows" and that should be carefully assessed so as not to be confused with visual hallucinations due to a psychiatric disorder (Lewis-Fernandez 1996).

Ethnocultural Values

Many values have been described that typify Puerto Ricans. Among them are *personalismo* (the need to relate to people and not to institutions), *confianza* (trust), *respeto* (respect), *verguenza* (shame), and *orgullo* (pride) (Rogler and Cooney 1984). *Familismo* (a family interdependence and loyalty), which reinforces cooperation over competition and expects the needs of the individual to be subordinate to the needs of the family, has been described as well (Ramos-McKay et al. 1988). Traditional gender roles have been coded into two frames: *marianismo* and *machismo*. *Marianismo* refers to the cultural belief that women are considered spiritually superior to men and are thus capable of enduring suffering better. *Machismo* refers to the cultural belief that the male is responsible for the welfare and honor of the family and should be the provider (Gomez 1982). These values are often affected by migration and social stressors, and the Puerto Rican mainland man's sense of masculinity may be undermined by discrimination, unemployment, and feelings of worthlessness (I. A. Canino and Canino 1980).

A study by Sommers and others (1993) that directly addressed the importance of these sociocultural influences on the behavior of Puerto Rican adolescents concluded that

Familism, a measure of the individual's expressed concern over family values rather than individual opportunities, was a consistent and direct contributor to the avoidance of deviance. This finding suggests that, in addition to respect and affection (family attachment), familial values, such as duty and obligation, are relevant to the cultural situation of adolescents. Acculturation was positively associated with participation in interpersonal violence and theft but lower acculturation was related to participation in illicit drug use. (p. 36)

In New York City Puerto Ricans, Bluestone and Vela (1982) described the cultural concept of time as it relates to their appointments, the cultural reactions to authority figures, and their difficulties modulating anger. They recommended the use of humor, metaphors, and proverbs and suggested that therapists should help their patients be more verbally assertive to deal with their new reality.

Puerto Rican families often emphasize the child's behavior both at home and in public. They underline the necessity of children to be obedient, to follow rules, and to conform in classroom settings (Zayas and Solari 1994). Relatedness and proper demeanor are highly valued, and parents prefer the child to be *educado* (well brought up), *amable* (polite and gentle), and *tranquilo, obediente,* and *respetuoso* (calm, obedient, and respectful). In contrast to Anglo-American mothers' concern with instilling in their toddlers an optimal balance of autonomy and relatedness, mainland Puerto Rican mothers focus on contextually appropriate levels of relatedness (R.L. Harwood et al. 1995). Puerto Rican parents also believe in social control based on strong family attachments and direct parental control based on discipline and coercion (Hagan 1989; Hirschi 1969; Paterson 1982).

Health-Seeking Behavior

Health-seeking behavior of Latinos in New York (Puerto Ricans were overrepresented in this group) indicated that acculturated Latinos were more likely than nonacculturated ones to use mental health services. Integration into the social network provided advice and referral information that made it more likely that they would seek services. In terms of types of mental health services, private therapists and prevention programs were reported as the most underused, whereas outpatient services and nonpsychiatric physicians were the most widely used (O. Rodriguez 1987).

Some studies have suggested that some Puerto Ricans in the United States avail themselves of spiritualist practices (*espiritismo*) as indigenous therapy, as a community support system, or as an outlet for the stressors caused by their economic and interpersonal circumstances (Garrison 1977; A. Harwood

1977). These practices have been described as being accessible, offering concrete solutions to problems, charging reasonable fees, communicating in the same language, and using the extended family in their healing practices (Lubchanski et al. 1970; Ruiz and Langrod 1976). Bird and Canino (1981) interviewed 50 Puerto Rican mothers in New York City and found that 24% had consulted a spiritualist about their child. They had taken the child because of behavior problems, academic difficulties, and sleep disturbances. The healers recommended taking herbal baths, reciting prayers, and wearing special articles of clothing.

In a recent study that assessed which psychologists treated minorities, Turner and Formaniak-Turner (1996) concluded that ethnic minority providers saw a larger proportion of ethnic minority patients than did non-Latino white providers. Those with an eclectic orientation as well as those with a cognitive-behavioral orientation saw more patients than did those with a psychodynamic or other theoretical orientation (Turner and Formaniak-Turner 1996).

Assessment

In describing the diagnosis and treatment for culturally diverse groups, DSM-IV-TR (American Psychiatric Association 2000) suggests a cultural formulation that consists of five principles:

1. The clinician should address the patient issues of cultural identity, which include cultural reference groups, language, cultural factors in development, and degree of involvement with the culture of origin and the host culture.
2. The clinician should assess the cultural explanations of the illness, which include idioms of distress and local illness categories, the meaning and severity of symptoms in relation to cultural norms, perceived causes and explanatory models, and health-seeking experiences and plans.
3. The clinician should address those cultural factors related to the patient's psychosocial environment and levels of functioning, which include social stressors and supports.
4. The clinician should be aware of the cultural elements of the clinician-patient relationship.
5. The clinician should conclude with an overall cultural assessment.

The following case example illustrates a patient with many cultural symptoms of distress and adjustment difficulties to a new culture and a new family.

Mrs. M, a 30-year-old Puerto Rican woman, finally had been referred to a bicultural, bilingual clinic by the family doctor of her 32-year-old husband after multiple unsuccessful attempts at treatment by a host of other specialists. She had been raised in a coastal town in Puerto Rico and had met her present husband during one of his trips to the island to visit some relatives. She married him and lived in Puerto Rico with him for 3 years. Mr. M was unable to adjust to her hometown and felt the same discrimination his parents had experienced in the United States. His poor Spanish language skills, his open support of his wife and help with her household chores, and his need for privacy were a constant source of conflict with his peers.

Mr. M had been raised in New York. His parents emigrated from Puerto Rico to New York when they were young. They were fluent in English and had attended public schools in New York. Mrs. M had agreed to live in New York to please her husband and to take advantage of the better opportunities for her children, Lisa, age 10, and Michael, age 8. She missed her family and hometown in Puerto Rico.

Mrs. M's chief complaint consisted of constant *preocupacion* (worry) about her children, *dolor de cerebro y en todo el cuerpo* (pain in the brain and in all her body), *mareos* (dizzy spells), and *miedo de la calle* (fear of the street). She felt that she had failed as a mother because her young daughter already liked to play too much with boys, and her son was too *presentao* and *ajentao* (outspoken and disrespectful and acted as if he were older). She perceived her husband's family as a bunch of *aprovechaos* and *abusaos* (taking advantage of people and situations), who had no *maneras* (manners) and were not *considerados* (considerate). All they thought about was competing and making money. They were so abrupt that she felt that they always were *coraje* (angry) with her. They did not know how to relax and *cosas cojer las con calma* (how to take things one at a time). They criticized her because she was never on time and she talked too much about personal things, even to strangers. They did not understand her inability to go on with life, to find a job, and to stop her complaining or her need to take a "martyr" role.

Mrs. M had no significant psychiatric history. Her family history included a mother who had had occasional *ataques* when she was stressed, but her many female friends in her community helped her with words of wisdom and herbal teas. Her father had been quite strict but a good man and provider. He had not been much of a friend to her mother and was not helpful at home or with the children. She had promised herself to find a man who would be her companion. This was one of the qualities about her husband that she liked best.

Mrs. M's headaches and dizzy spells initially had concerned the family, and they told her to see the family doctor, who recommended a series of expensive tests and multiple referrals to specialists. Nothing was found. She then sought help for her fear and *tristeza* (sadness). Multiple antidepressive and antianxiety medications were recommended. She would report an immediate positive effect for a couple of days and then would report either side effects or that the medicine just did not resolve her problems. She felt uncomfortable informing her doctors that the treatments were not working (after all, they were supposed to know everything and could be offended if she told them the truth). Mr. M, who had attended some of those interviews, was always surprised at her willingness to please and "be a good patient." He also felt that she overreported her symptoms and made them sound worse than they really were. During one of her interviews, Mrs. M reported a lack of sleep and poor appetite and was given a diagnosis of a depressive disorder. This diagnosis concerned her, even though she later admitted that she could not say "no" to the doctor's insistent questions about the subject. She actually did not express these symptoms unless she was worried about her children regarding a specific incident. The distress symptoms never lasted more than a few days.

After a very careful psychiatric evaluation, it was determined that Mrs. M was expressing many cultural symptoms of distress and having adjustment difficulties to a new culture and a new family. On closer inspection, she had no problem leaving the house in her hometown in Puerto Rico, and many of her physical symptoms abated when she visited the island. She felt much better when she spoke on the telephone with her sisters in Puerto Rico. They acknowledged her distress and commented on the personal sacrifices she was making for her children and husband. They also told her that "she was a great mother and wife; that she was just not appreciated by her new family; one day they would recognize her sacrifices."

Clearly, this is a case of cultural misperceptions from both families. Mrs. M's new family was well-intentioned, caring, resourceful, and patient. They truly wanted her to be independent, happy, and self-reliant. They also felt that her son was appropriately assertive and that her daughter was learning how to treat boys in the future, by mixing with them from a young age. They felt that both children were developing good independent skills but were concerned that Mrs. M's overprotectiveness would not prepare them for the harsh life in the city. They perceived Mrs. M as too traditional, too sensitive, too accommodating, and too acquiescent. They felt that she should express herself openly and assertively with her doctor and other authority figures.

The clinic offered a family intervention in which the therapist took on the role of a "cultural broker and translator" by discussing the power of misperceptions and underlining the strengths of both cultures. All the family members were of Puerto Rican descent but had different levels of acculturation, different contextual experiences, different expectations, and different idiomatic expressions of distress. The therapist helped the family learn from one another and helped them to clarify the differences between being assertive and aggressive, expressive and outspoken, well mannered and acquiescent, and concerned and overprotective. The somatic expressions of distress were integrated as an equally important communication to seek help and attention. The therapist discussed the equally difficult time of the husband in Puerto Rico and suggested that it would benefit him and his family to learn more about the cultural patterns in her hometown. Both groups were informed of the dynamic and fast changes in cultural norms on both the island and the mainland. If they looked closely enough, they would find that many cultural traditions had changed in the island, with some sections of the population acting quite "American." They also would discover that some pockets of Puerto Ricans in the United States still held fast to traditions that were no longer practiced in Puerto Rico. They were advised that it was worth learning a bicultural language that would allow them to move in both changing worlds.

CONCLUSIONS

Mainland Puerto Ricans have a complex history of migration and labor participation in the United States. They live in a variety of different communities and are at different levels of acculturation. They may be bilingual or monolingual in Spanish or in English, and they may still have relatives in Puerto Rico. Some of them have married Puerto Ricans, whereas others have married other ethnic groups. They share some similar values and, like all groups, have intragroup differences.

Despite some methodological limitations, research to address the mental health profiles of Puerto Ricans both on the island and in the mainland United States has been increasing. Preliminary findings suggest areas of sociocultural strengths as well as areas of vulnerability and risk. This chapter discusses some of the findings in depression, substance use, and somatization as examples of the importance of considering sociodemographic and cultural variables in the interpretation of the results.

Similar caution is suggested when discussing clinical guidelines that address issues of language and idioms of distress. A review of terms used by some members of the culture, perhaps the less acculturated ones or those less exposed to current mental health resources, to communicate stress or symptoms is offered to avoid clinician-patient misunderstandings. *Ataques de nervios* is mentioned as an example, and a clinical vignette is provided in the previous section to illustrate the clinical relevance of these principles.

Finally, in this chapter, we address the intracultural complexities that are often encountered in families at different levels of acculturation and with different socialization experiences. The constantly changing and complex nature of idioms of distress, symptomatic presentation, and patterns of health-seeking behavior and delivery pose many questions to researchers. Clinically, this chapter offers mental health workers the challenge of differentiating among sociocultural, biological, and psychological etiological theories of disorder and the constant search for treatment approaches that are specific and effective.

REFERENCES

American Psychiatric Association: Diagnostic and Statistical Manual of Mental Disorders, 3rd Edition. Washington, DC, American Psychiatric Association, 1980

American Psychiatric Association: Diagnostic and Statistical Manual of Mental Disorders, 4th Edition, Text Revision. Washington, DC, American Psychiatric Association, 2000

Anthony JC, Helzer JE: Syndromes of drug abuse and dependence, in Psychiatric Disorders in America. Edited by Robins L, Regier D. New York, Free Press, 1991, pp 116–154

Bird H, Canino I: The socio-psychiatry of espiritismo: findings of a study in psychiatric populations of Puerto Ricans and other Hispanic children. J Am Acad Child Adolesc Psychiatry 20:725–740, 1981

Bluestone H, Vela RM: Transcultural aspects in the psychotherapy of Puerto Rican poor in New York City. J Am Acad Pychoanal 10:269–282, 1982

Canino G, Bird H, Shrout P, et al: The prevalence of alcohol abuse and/or dependence in Puerto Rico, in Health and Behavior: Research Agenda for Hispanics (Series 1). Edited by Gaviria M, Arana J. Chicago, The University of Illinois at Chicago, 1987a, pp 127–144

Canino G, Bird H, Shrout P, et al: The prevalence of specific psychiatric disorders in Puerto Rico. Arch Gen Psychiatry 44:727–735, 1987b

Canino G, Burnam A, Caetano R: The prevalence of alcohol abuse and/or dependence in two Hispanic communities, in Alcoholism in North America, Europe, and Asia. Edited by Helzer JE, Canino GJ. New York, Oxford University Press, 1992, pp 131–158

Canino G, Anthony JC, Freeman D, et al: Drug abuse and illicit drug use in Puerto Rico. Am J Public Health 83:194–200, 1993

Canino IA, Canino G: Impact of stress on the Puerto Rican family: treatment considerations. Am J Orthopsychiatry 50:535–541, 1980

Canino IA, Rubio-Stipec M, Canino G, et al: Functional somatic symptoms: a cross-ethnic comparison. Am J Orthopsychiatry 62:605–612, 1992

Cortez DE, Rogler LH: Health status and acculturation among Puerto Ricans in New York City. Journal of Gender, Culture and Health 1:267–276, 1996

Escobar JI, Gomez J, Tuason VB: Depressive phenomenology in North and South American patients. Am J Psychiatry 140:47–51, 1983

Garrison V: Doctor, espiritista, or psychiatrist? Help seeking behavior in a Puerto Rican neighborhood in New York City. Med Anthropol 1:164–185, 1977

Gomez AG: The Puerto Rican American, in Cross-Cultural Psychiatry. Edited by Gaw A. Littleton, MA, John Wright–PSG Publishing, 1982, pp 109–136

Guarnaccia PJ, Rodriguez O: Concepts of culture and their role in the development of culturally competent mental health services. Hispanic Journal of Behavioral Sciences 18:419–443, 1996

Guarnaccia P, Rubio-Stipec M, Canino G: *Ataques de nervios* in the Puerto Rican Diagnostic Interview Schedule: the impact of cultural categories on psychiatric epidemiology. Cult Med Psychiatry 13:257–295, 1989

Guarnaccia PJ, Good BJ, Kleinman A: A critical review of epidemiological studies of Puerto Rican mental health. Am J Psychiatry 147:1449–1456, 1990

Hagan J: Structural Criminology. New Brunswick, NJ, Rutgers University Press, 1989

Hakuta K, Garcia EE: Bilingualism and education. Am Psychol 44:374–379, 1989

Harwood A: Rx: Spiritist as Needed. New York, Wiley, 1977

Harwood RL, Miller JL, Irizarry NL: Culture and Attachment: Perceptions of the Child in Context. New York, Guilford, 1995

Helzer J, Canino G: Comparative analysis of alcoholism in ten cultural regions, in Alcoholism in North America, Europe, and Asia. Edited by Helzer JE, Canino GJ. New York, Oxford University Press, 1992, pp 289–308

Hirschi T: Causes of Delinquency. Berkeley, University of California Press, 1969

Lewis-Fernandez R: Cultural formulation of psychiatric diagnosis: Case No 02, diagnosis and treatment of nervios and ataques in a female Puerto Rican migrant. Cult Med Psychiatry 20:155–163, 1996

Lubchanski I, Egri G, Stokes J: Puerto Rican spiritualists view mental illness: the faith healer as a paraprofessional. Am J Psychiatry 127:312–331, 1970

Mendoza FS, Ventura SJ, Valdez RB, et al: Selected measures of health status for Mexican-American, mainland Puerto Ricans, and Cuban-American children. JAMA 265:227–232, 1991

Mezzich JE, Raab ES: Depressive symptomatology across the Americas. Arch Gen Psychiatry 27:818–823, 1980

Moscicki EK, Locke BZ, Rae DS, et al: Depressive symptoms among Mexican Americans: the Hispanic Health and Nutrition Examination Survey. Am J Epidemiol 130:348–360, 1989

Ortiz A, Medina-Mora ME: Research on drug abuse in Mexico, in Epidemiology of Drug Abuse and Issues Among Native American Populations: Community Epidemiology Work Group Proceedings, December 1987 (Contract No 271-87-8321). Washington, DC, U.S. Government Printing Office, 1988

Paterson GR: Coercive Family Process. Eugene, OR, Castalia, 1982

Ramos-McKay JM, Comas-Diaz L, Rivera LA: Puerto Ricans, in Clinical Guidelines in Cross-Cultural Mental Health. Edited by Comas-Diaz L, Griffith EEH. New York, Wiley, 1988, pp 204–232

Rivera-Batiz FL, Santiago C: Puerto Ricans in the United States: A Changing Reality. Washington, DC, The National Puerto Rican Coalition, 1995

Rodriguez C: Puerto Ricans Born in the United States. Boston, MA, Unwin Hyman, 1989

Rodriguez O: Hispanics and Human Services: Help Seeking in the Inner City (Hispanic Research Center, Monograph 14). New York, Fordham University Press, 1987

Rogler LH, Cooney RS: Puerto Rican Families in New York City: Intergenerational Processes. Maplewood, NJ, Waterfront Press, 1984

Rogler LH, Cortez DE, Malgady RG: The mental health relevance of idioms of distress: anger and perceptions of injustice among New York Puerto Ricans. J Nerv Ment Dis 182:327–330, 1994

Rosenwaike I: Mortality differentials among persons born in Cuba, Mexico and Puerto Rico residing in the United States, 1979–1981. Am J Public Health 77:603–606, 1987

Rubio-Stipec M, Shrout P, Bird H, et al: Symptom scales of the Diagnostic Interview Schedule: factor results in Hispanic and Anglo samples. J Consult Clin Psychol 1:30–34, 1989

Rubio-Stipec M, Canino G, Robin LN, et al: The somatization schedule of the Composite International Diagnostic Interview (CIDI): the use of the probe flow chart in 17 different countries. International Journal of Methods in Psychiatric Research 3(2):129–136, 1993

Ruiz P, Langrod J: The role of folk healers in community mental health services. Community Ment Health J 12:392–398, 1976

Santiago AM: Patterns of Puerto Rican segregation and mobility (Special Issue: Puerto Rican Poverty and Labor Markets). Hispanic Journal of Behavioral Sciences 14:107–133, 1992

Senior C, Watkins DO: Toward a balance sheet of Puerto Rican migration, in Status of Puerto Rico: Selected Background Studies (Prepared for the U.S.–Puerto Rico Commission on the Status of Puerto Rico). Washington, DC, U.S. Government Printing Office, 1966

Sommers I, Fagan J, Baskin D: Socio-cultural influences on the explanation of delinquency for Puerto Rican youths. Hispanic Journal of Behavioral Sciences 15:36–62, 1993

Stevens-Arroyo A, Diaz-Stevens AM: Puerto Ricans in the States: a struggle for identity, in The Minority Report: An Introduction to Racial, Ethnic and Gender Relations, 2nd Edition. Edited by Dworkin AG, Dworkin RJ. New York, College Publishing, Holt, Rinehart & Winston, 1982, pp 196–232

Swerdlow M: Nervios and community care: a case study of Puerto Rican psychiatric patients in New York City. Cult Med Psychiatry 16:217–235, 1992

Therrien M, Ramirez RR: The Hispanic Population in the United States. March 2000, Current Population Reports, Series P-20: Population Characteristics, No. 535. Washington, DC, U.S. Bureau of the Census, February 2000. Available at: http://www.census.gov/population/socdemo/hispanic/p20-535/p20-535.pdf

Turner CB, Formaniak-Turner B: Who treats minorities? Cultural Diversity and Mental Health 2:175–182, 1996

Vega WA, Kolody B, Aguilar-Gaxiola S, et al: Lifetime prevalence of DSM-III-R psychiatric disorders among urban and rural Mexican Americans in California. Arch Gen Psychiatry 55:771–778, 1998

Vega WA, Kolody B, Aguilar-Gaxiola S, et al: Gaps in service utilization by Mexican Americans with mental health problems. Am J Psychiatry 156:928–934, 1999

Vera M, Alegria M, Freeman D, et al: Depressive symptoms among Puerto Rican Island poor compared with residents in the New York City area. Am J Epidemiol 134:502–510, 1991

Wasserman GA, Brunelli SA, Rauh VA, et al: The cultural context of child rearing in three groups of urban minority mothers (Chapter 7), in Puerto Rican Women and Children: Issues in Health, Growth, and Development. Edited by Lamberty G, Garcia-Coll C. New York, Plenum, 1994

Wells KB, Hough RL, Golding JM, et al: Which Mexican Americans underutilize health services? Am J Psychiatry 144:918–922, 1987

Zayas LH, Solari F: Early childhood socialization in Hispanic families: context, culture, and practice implications. Professional Psychology: Research and Practice 25:200–206, 1994

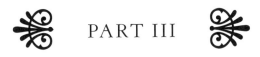

PART III

Special Issues and Populations

CHAPTER 12

Domestic Violence in the Latino Population

Michael A. Rodriguez, M.D., M.P.H.

Heidi M. Bauer, M.D., M.P.H., M.S.

Yvette Flores-Ortiz, Ph.D.

THE PURPOSE OF THIS chapter is to provide a framework for understanding domestic violence and for responding to the problem with Latino patients. Although extensive research on domestic violence among Latinos has yet to be conducted, available data suggest that domestic violence is a significant problem in the lives of many Latinas. Latinas have unique cultural values and face many social, economic, and acculturation forces that may affect the occurrence of partner abuse or interfere with an abused woman's ability to seek help.

Domestic violence, also referred to as partner or wife abuse, is a pattern of coercive behaviors that involves physical abuse or the threat of physical abuse. It also may include repeated psychological abuse, sexual assault, progressive social isolation, deprivation, intimidation, or economic coercion. Domestic violence is violence perpetrated by adults or adolescents against their intimate partners in current or former dating, marital, or cohabiting couples of heterosexuals, gay men, lesbians, bisexuals, and transgendered people.

In this chapter, we review the literature on domestic violence among Latinos and provide an overview of Latino cultural norms and values, as well as social and acculturation forces that may affect domestic violence. Because 95% of the reported assaults on spouses or ex-spouses are committed by men against women, we focus primarily on abuse of Latinas. Data from focus groups of abused Latina immigrant women are presented in an effort to understand the experiences, perceptions, and expectations of women. Finally, we offer specific recommendations for the evaluation and treatment of Latina victims of domestic violence.

THEORETICAL, SOCIAL, AND CULTURAL ISSUES

Numerous frameworks have been developed to understand wife abuse. Some disciplines view domestic violence as a manifestation of individual psychiatric disorders (either the abused, the abuser, or both), whereas others view abuse as a product of dysfunctional family dynamics. In contrast to these theories, the feminist framework for understanding the occurrence of domestic violence centers on the primacy of gender and gender-based power inequities in society (Bograd 1988; Dobash and Dobash 1979; Kurz 1989). Implications for solutions of marital abuse thus lie in the empowerment of women and fundamental changes in social and economic institutions that perpetuate gender inequities. One limitation of this model is its limited explanatory power in relation to abuse among gay and lesbian couples and the abuse of men by women.

In addition to gender considerations, an analysis of cultural, social, and economic forces that play a role in domestic violence is critical (Lockhart 1987; Wyatt 1994). Although the problem of domestic violence cuts across all class and racial/ethnic groups, it is important to consider how social and cultural forces may operate to initiate, discourage, or perpetuate domestic violence against women. In addition, these forces may affect the willingness and ability of abused women to seek care and respond to interventions. In particular, cultural values that emphasize female passivity may decrease abused women's willingness to assert their independence and seek help. Values that emphasize family unity may be protective against the abuse of wives but also may inhibit victims from seeking help from social institutions outside the community (Ho 1990; Lin and Tan 1994). Social forces such as poverty, sexism, and racism have a profound effect on domestic violence in minority populations. Understanding the social context not only is important for the clinician but also may facilitate recovery for both victim and perpetrator (Flores-Ortiz 1992).

Several caveats must be considered when making generalizations about Latino culture or class. First, it is important to clarify the distinctions between cultural and social forces and understand their interactions. Constructing inaccurate conceptions that Latinos are inherently prone to violence because of cultural values rather than social forces risks blaming the subgroup culture for problems derived from their social context. The gender oppression and glorification and sexualization of violence in American culture also must be considered in framing the origins of subgroup behavior. Second, generalizations must make room for diversity among Latinos, which is in part based on differences in religion, class background, urban versus rural setting, and level of acculturation, but also is based on differences among families and individuals that transcend cultural norms. Third, cultural norms are dynamic and adaptable. Norms change in response to acculturation, changing systems of economics, technology, and communication. In summary, generalizations may be helpful in beginning to understand a patient's social context, but ultimately his or her experience and perceptions are informed by a multitude of factors.

ABUSED WOMEN AND
THE HEALTH CARE SYSTEM

Domestic violence is one of the most serious social and public health issues of our time. Every year, an estimated 2–4 million women in the United States are abused by an intimate partner. Government research has shown that one-third of all women murdered in this country are murdered by their current or former husbands or boyfriends (Bureau of Justice Statistics 1994). Abused women make up a significant proportion of various patient populations (Abbot et al. 1995; Gin et al. 1991; Hamberger et al. 1992; Helton et al. 1987; McCauley et al. 1995; McFarlane et al. 1992; Rath et al. 1989). Furthermore, women who are battered use medical services more frequently than do women who are not abused because of increased physical injuries, medical problems, and somatization (Bergman and Brismar 1991; Cascardi et al. 1992; Drossman et al. 1990; Koss and Heslet 1992; McCauley et al. 1995; Plichta 1992). Despite the significant health implications of domestic violence, health providers often fail to identify and assist victims, even when signs and symptoms are present (Hamberger et al. 1992; Warshaw 1989). Furthermore, abused women are more likely to be dissatisfied with their medical care compared with nonabused women (Plichta et al. 1996).

Abused women also are at increased risk for psychological stress and psychiatric disorders (Browne 1993; Plichta 1992). In particular, several studies have shown that battered women have higher rates of depression, anxiety disorders, substance abuse (including alcohol), and suicide attempts than do nonbattered women (Amaro et al. 1990; Bergman and Brismar 1991; Cascardi et al. 1992; McCauley et al. 1995; Neff et al. 1995; Saunders et al. 1993).

The *battered woman's syndrome* is a commonly used term for the psychological sequelae of repeated abuse and violence (Walker 1979). This concept incorporates ideas about learned helplessness and characterizes victims as passive, hopeless, and developing low self-esteem as a result of the abuse. Another way of understanding the psychological responses of victims is through the diagnostic construct of posttraumatic stress disorder (PTSD) (Browne 1993). It is argued that repeated violence and abuse may result in typical symptoms of PTSD, including fear, flashbacks, denial, avoidance, loss of memory, anxiety, and hypervigilance. Ultimately, these constructs may provide only limited guidance given the diversity of experiences and psychological adaptations of abuse survivors.

Abused women face many barriers to care (Leung and Smith 1994). Many are socially isolated or lack adequate information about available social and community resources. Women who are poor or economically controlled may face financial barriers to certain services. The lack of linguistically and culturally appropriate services may deter many women minorities, immigrants, and women who speak limited English. Immigrants, in particular, often lack knowledge about their legal rights and the available resources; also, many may fear deportation if they are undocumented (Jang 1994). Many abused women are reluctant to identify themselves because of shame or fear of reprisal from the abusive partner. Others may be in denial or inhibited by a sense of helplessness. Still others may be reluctant to seek help out of loyalty to the abusive partner or a desire to keep the family together.

Even in situations in which abused women want to reach out for help, they are often confronted with insensitivity and judgmental attitudes on the part of providers. The medical system in particular tends to have an individualistic focus on pathophysiology rather than psychological or social problems (Warshaw 1989). Provider barriers to identifying and treating victims of partner abuse include time constraints, lack of adequate training, fear of offending patients, and personal discomfort and sense of powerlessness (Brown et al. 1993; Ferris and Tudiver 1992; Sugg and Inui 1992). One explanation for some of these problems is that many health care institutions lack staff policies, resources, and educational curriculum that focus on battered women. Given the high prevalence of domestic violence, the seriousness of both physical and psychological outcomes, and the myriad barriers to care faced by abused women, it is critical that mental health providers respond affirmatively to make care more accessible, sensitive, and culturally appropriate.

DOMESTIC VIOLENCE AND THE LATINO COMMUNITY

Research on the prevalence of the social and cultural factors that affect the occurrence of marital violence among Latinos is limited. A few studies have sampled Latinos in sufficient numbers to estimate prevalence, but rates have varied significantly because of differences in measurements and sample populations. Furthermore, although some work has measured acculturation, instruments on domestic violence that reliably measure cultural beliefs and norms are scarce. Despite this lack of research, identifiable cultural and social factors may be relevant to understanding the occurrence of domestic violence in the Latino community and abused women's response.

Prevalence of Marital Violence Among Latinos

Because of differences in measurements and sample populations, the prevalence of domestic violence among Latinos varies substantially. According to data from the 1985 National Family Violence Survey, English-speaking Latino couples reported markedly higher rates of marital violence (17%) compared with non-Latino white couples (11%) (Straus and Smith 1989). According to a survey of Los Angeles, California, households, the lifetime rates of spousal violence were nearly equivalent for Mexican Americans and non-Latino whites (20.0% and 21.6%, respectively) (Sorenson and Telles 1991). On the basis of data from the National Crime Victimization Survey, the Bureau of Justice Statistics (1994) reported that Hispanic and non-Hispanic white women had about the same annual rate of violence attributable to intimates—6 per 1,000 women. The fact that this rate is significantly lower than rates found by other researchers may be because of the focus of the research on activity that is specifically defined as criminal. The literature of 2000 reports history of intimate partner abuse among Latinos to be 10.0% (Bauer and Rodriguez 1995). In general, higher rates of domestic violence are strongly associated with younger age, low income, unemployment, and urbanicity.

Another survey of several Latino subgroups found that the prevalence of domestic violence ranged from 2.5% to 20.4%, compared with 9.9% for whites (Kantor et al. 1994). However, Neff et al. (1995) found that the rate was 30% for Mexican Americans, compared with 26% for whites. Both of these studies examined the role of social and psychological factors. In general, domestic violence was correlated with a greater acceptance of interpersonal violence (Kantor et al. 1994), sex role traditionalism, and economic stressors (Neff et al. 1995). When these factors were controlled in multivariate analyses, ethnicity had no independent effect on the rate of domestic violence. Overall, the rates of partner abuse among Latinos vary from 2.5% to 30% depending on the population sampled and measurements of violence and abuse. Although many questions about the epidemiology of marital violence in Latino communities remain unanswered, it is clear that wife abuse is a serious problem affecting many Latinas.

Latino Cultural Values and Domestic Violence

Despite the diversity among Latino communities, families, and individuals, there appear to be certain common values. Allocentrism and famillilism are considered important values that serve to structure the collectivism and interdependency with Latino culture, whereas interpersonal interactions are guided by norms of *simpatía* (preference for positive interpersonal relationships characterized by politeness and avoidance of conflict) and *respeto* (respect) (Marín and Marín 1991; Molina et al. 1994). Culturally constructed gender roles, particularly within the family, are an important feature of Latino culture and may play a role in the occurrence of and response to domestic violence.

Familismo

Familismo (the strong identification with and attachment, loyalty, and duty to the nuclear and extended family) may operate as a protective factor or source of help for abused Latinas. The social support provided by extended family, the Catholic church, and the collectivism of the Latino community potentially serve as a buffer from social and economic stresses. Extended family members not only provide material support but also serve as a social control mechanism within the community. The strength and pride of the Latino community may serve to discourage domestic violence.

On the other hand, the value of *familismo* may present barriers to women seeking outside help because it increases the stigma of divorce, creates an expectation that problems are kept within the family, and may increase the tolerance to abuse for the sake of family dignity (Zambrano 1985). In a qualitative study involving diverse ethnic groups, the desire to keep the family together was an important cultural force that interfered with help seeking for many abused women (Sorenson 1996). Gondolf et al. (1988) studied shelter residents and found that compared with white and black women, Latinas were the least likely to have sought help through a friend, minister, or social service agency. This finding may be related to the strong value of kinship and family dependency among Latinos.

Loyalty to the husband, beliefs that children need to live with their father, and the stigma of divorce may lead to greater acceptance of violence and mistreatment among abused Latinas. Furthermore, these cultural values play a role in willingness to seek care in that the barriers to ending the relationship are often the same barriers to seeking help or confiding in a health care professional.

Machismo

Traditionally, Latino families were seen as having rigid patriarchal structures in which *machismo* (the cultural belief that the male is responsible for the welfare and honor of the family and should be the provider) and female submissiveness were key variables in explaining family dynamics. Although it is argued that *machismo* and the Latino patriarchy predispose husbands to using physical force against their wives, it also can be asserted that Latino men who abuse their power and authority through domestic violence lose respect in the larger Latino community (Mirande 1985).

Few studies have attempted to understand the relation between gender roles and domestic violence among Latinos. However, one study of abused Latinas indicated that power imbalances and the lack of mutuality in the marital relationship were correlated with higher rates of abuse (Perilla et al. 1994). In addition, these researchers found that the abuser's frequency of alcohol abuse and intoxication was correlated with violence.

Marianismo

The cultural construct of *marianismo,* or the long-suffering mother, encourages women to be docile, quiet, self-sacrificing, and stoic (Martinez 1988; Panitz et al. 1983). In this construct, husband-wife relationships are often characterized by control and dependency in that women are expected to be submissive and obedient in relation to their spouse. Latinas are essential to family functioning and the transmission of cultural values; as a reward for this hard work and obedience, mothers are revered within the culture (Mirande and Enriquez 1979; Staples and Mirande 1989).

Culturally influenced gender role expectations may significantly impede abused Latinas' ability and willingness to seek help or end the relationship. Latinas have been found to be more tolerant of abuse and to perceive fewer types of behavior as being abusive (Torres 1991). Gondolf et al. (1988) found that Latinas have greater tolerance of abuse and devotion to keeping their families together than do white and black women and concluded that Latinas appear to be "bound by a norm of loyal motherhood" that kept them in abusive relationships.

Simpatía, Respeto, and Confianza

Simpatía, a cultural script derived from allocentric values, emphasizes behavior that promotes smooth and pleasant social interactions through empathy, respect, and a certain amount of conformity (Marín and Marín 1991; Martinez 1988). It also describes a general tendency to avoid interpersonal conflict and confrontation and expression of uncomfortable emotions. Latina women's modesty and indirect styles of communication may discourage abused women from discussing their concerns publicly (Ginorio and Reno 1986). The *simpatía* of women may make them less likely to be assertive or to complain of their situation.

The distance between Latinas and health care providers can interfere with open communication about domestic violence on the part of Latinas. Many Latinas are sensitive to provider behavior, class and social status differences, and cultural sensitivity, which create distance in the patient-provider relationship. Many Latinas desire *respeto* (mutual respect) from health care providers.

Confianza denotes the constellation of trust, confidentiality, comfort, and safety that is critical for creating rapport between Latina patients and health care professionals. Many Latina patients prefer a relationship that is warm, friendly, and personal. Abused Latinas may benefit from health care providers who are patient, attentive, compassionate, and trustworthy.

Latino Socioeconomic Factors and Domestic Violence

Social and economic forces likely play a significant role in increased rates of domestic violence in Latinas. It is commonly accepted that economic deprivation can create intrafamilial conflict and lead to higher rates of violence (Straus and Smith 1989). Compared with non-Hispanic whites, Latinos tend to have lower levels of formal education, greater levels of unemployment, and higher rates of poverty (Garcia 1991). Evidence that these stresses affect the rates of marital violence among Latinos comes from several studies that found a confounding effect of socioeconomic factors on rates of partner violence (Kantor et al. 1994; Neff et al. 1995). In addition, abused Latinas are more likely to report subjective economic stress compared with nonabused Latinas (Perilla et al. 1994). The lack of economic resources or opportunities also may serve as an impediment to help-seeking for or leaving an abusive relationship for Latinas.

Racial/Ethnic Discrimination

Racism and racial/ethnic discrimination are another source of stress for Latinos in this country. Opinion polls have shown that most Americans hold pejorative views of Latinos (Asbury 1993). Although this pervasive racism takes a tremendous psychological toll on its victims, it is the institutionalized racism that operates to create a social situation that denies Latinos access to many economic and educational opportunities. Clearly, these socially oppressive forces affect the experiences of both immigrant and United States–born Latinos.

The experience of racism may serve as a barrier to help seeking because abused Latinas may fear that their partners will be treated badly by authorities because of their ethnicity. In addition, many minorities feel alienated from social and legal services. Furthermore, the lack of culturally relevant health settings and culturally sensitive providers decreases use of health services (Williams and Becker 1994; Woodward et al. 1992). The sense of marginalization based on ethnic differences serves as an important barrier to seeking care and attaining a trusting relationship with a provider.

Immigration and Acculturation

The powerful effect of immigration and acculturation on Latinas must be considered in understanding Latino experiences. Many Latino immigrants arrive with the expectation of a better life, which eventually gives way to the realities of prejudice, language barriers, and poverty (Ruiz 1977). This disillusion and culture shock create incredible stress within immigrant communities. Furthermore, acculturation can cause important personal intrafamilial problems because minority groups tend to incorporate the negative value judgments of the dominant culture, which results in lowered self-esteem and the potential for increased conflict (Curtis 1990).

Cultural transitions may create personal and intrafamilial problems, which may lead to the use of violence. For example, family conflict may arise because of uneven acculturation of family members, particularly of spouses (Jalali 1988). On the basis of her research with abusive Latino families, Flores-Ortiz (1992) developed the idea of "cultural freezing," in which families develop rigid, stereotyped values and behaviors as a result of a difficult acculturation process. Freezing may occur when a woman's desire for greater independence is construed as a failure of family unity and thus a failure of her gendered and culturally prescribed duties. The man or family may feel entitled to punish her in the interest of keeping the family together. Because of the socialization of Latinas, they feel compelled to remain in the abusive relationship and preserve the family unit. Although these forces are not universal for Latino immigrants, they may play a significant role in contributing to marital violence. These assertions are supported by studies that compared foreign-born and United States–born Latinos and found higher rates of domestic violence for United States–born Latinos (Kantor et al. 1994; Sorenson and Telles 1991). In addition, Perilla et al. (1994) found that the rate of abuse among Latino couples increased with increasing economic contributions of the woman, indicating that abusive husbands are threatened by the disruption of traditional gender roles and resort to physical violence to regain lost authority.

In some cases, immigrant women are dependent on their husbands for citizenship, thus preventing them from seeking help if they are being abused. In fact, the threat of deportation or withholding information regarding citizenship is an often-used form of abuse (Jang 1994). Although local law enforcement authorities have no duty to enforce federal immigration laws, undocumented women face the fear that they will be reported if they seek criminal or civil legal assistance. In addition, these women typically are ineligible for public assistance and face employment barriers that perpetuate their economic dependence on the abusive spouse.

Language Barriers

Many Latinas face significant language barriers in seeking medical, social, or legal services (Woodward et al. 1992). Inadequate interpretation or translation compromises patient care, interferes with the diagnostic power of the interview, impairs patient education, decreases compliance and follow-up, and often results in overall patient dissatisfaction (Woloshin et al. 1995). Also, subtleties of culture are lost, which leads to misunderstanding and frustration (Haffner 1992).

In the case of abused Latinas, communication is a key issue. The common practice of using family members to interpret in clinical settings is inappropriate because it compromises confidentiality and makes the victim less likely to disclose her abuse. Even the use of interpreters can be problematic because it involves a third person and creates distance between the patient and the provider.

IMPLICATIONS FOR EVALUATION AND TREATMENT

Key to any intervention with battered Latinas and their partners is the development of trust. The health care provider should initiate inquiry through gentle, supportive, and nonjudgmental questions. The treatment provider may need to address the abused patient's concerns directly (e.g., confidentiality, whether disclosure will lead to deportation, police reports). Clear, useful information about resources and direct referrals facilitated by the provider are essential. The most helpful way to overcome the patient's reluctance to disclose or discuss abuse is by making her feel understood, supported, and valued.

The goal of individual and family interventions for Latinos who face domestic violence is to seek in the culture the family resources and solutions to end the abuse, exploitation, and pain. The key to treating domestic violence in a culturally integrated way is to offer services for the family. Whether the services are medical, psychological, or social and directed at the woman or the perpetrator, they must have a commitment to address the needs of the entire family (Flores-Ortiz 1992; Flores-Ortiz et al. 1994).

Identification

Domestic violence and its psychiatric and medical sequelae are sufficiently prevalent to justify routine screening of all female patients in mental health settings. Because some women may not initially recognize themselves as "abused," the provider should routinely ask all women direct, specific questions about abuse. It is important to screen in a safe environment, with a nonthreatening, nonjudgmental manner. Patients may respond better if questions are direct, specific, and easy to understand. For example, "Has your partner physically hurt or threatened you?" or "Many people come in with symptoms like yours and often they are related to someone hurting them. Is this what happened (is happening) to you?" With a rapport of trust, support, and compassion, early recognition and intervention may reduce the morbidity and mortality that results from domestic violence.

Evaluation

The first step in the treatment of domestic violence is through evaluation, paying particular attention to lethality, the likelihood that a homicide may occur. This safety assessment can be accomplished through questions about immediate danger, history of abuse and its duration, drug or alcohol abuse, and whether weapons have been used or if they are present in the household. It is important to explore types of safety strategies used (e.g., how the woman protects herself, whether she has sought assistance for the violence and from whom, whether she has tried to leave in the past and what happened). Other issues to assess include the degree of the abuser's control over the patient (e.g., threats, restricting freedom, financial), effects of domestic violence on mental and physical health, and effects on children. Frequently, it is in everyone's best interests if the couple temporarily separates. When the provider suggests separation as an effort to save the family and protect everyone, the recommendation, even when enforced legally, is more likely to be accepted and followed through by the family.

It is important to assess the victim's psychological response to abuse, such as minimization, denial, guilt, sadness, grief, fear, or anxiety. The patient's views and attitudes toward how the abuse has affected her, how she copes, and what she would like to see happen to herself and her family are important. Attribution of causality and sense of responsibility are other psychological issues to assess. The identification of concurrent psychiatric problems in all family members also is essential for treatment planning. The clinician should recognize that substance abuse may be a form of self-medication. During evaluation, any psychiatric symptoms should be assumed to be the consequence of abuse rather than preexisting.

It is also important to evaluate the socioeconomic and cultural context of the family, including the woman's economic viability and family member's levels of acculturation and cultural connection. Particularly helpful at this stage is integrated case management, which includes the identification of social and cultural needs. Psychological evaluations of children and adults can help determine the need for individual therapy and identify child abuse or neglect (Flores-Ortiz 1992).

The national origins of patients; their history of migration; reasons for migration; and postmigration experiences, including degree of disruption to family patterns, should be assessed to determine the degree of psychosocial stressors that the family has faced. The family's sources of acculturative stress, social supports, and resources should be determined to identify options for safety and factors for potential abuse. Likewise, such information will bring forth the cultural uniqueness of the individual and family and will help determine appropriate, culturally congruent interventions.

It is also important to assess the patient's own definition of violence and the degree of cultural freezing that may interfere with help seeking. Finally, an assessment of the patient's own perception of barriers and pressures to help seeking is useful in determining the degree of support she will need to follow through with treatment recommendations and referrals. Latinas often require a team approach with strong case management and personal contact before treatment is obtained.

Intervention

The primary goal of all interventions is to end the violence while maintaining respect for self-determination and autonomy. It is important to examine the individual, interpersonal, social, and political roots of violence to promote strategies that heal, empower, and offer new ways of coping and problem solving. To that end, multiple modalities of treatment can and should be made available to Latinas, including support groups for battered women, social services to address economic and familial pressures, and individual and family counseling (Flores-Ortiz 1998). Whatever the intervention, a central objective should be the establishment of a safety plan and safeguards for the protection of children. Moreover, as a result of federal and state policies, particular sensitivity is needed regarding the needs of undocumented women.

The health care provider must be sensitive, be responsive, and focus on building rapport and trust. This is facilitated by conveying messages of support because women who have lived with violence often need extra support before they can become their own advocates. Providing information about the frequency of domestic violence and the effects of domestic violence also is useful. This information includes the cycle of domestic violence, how it generally continues and increases over time, and how it can have long-term damaging effects on children in the home. It is also important to note that domestic violence is a crime, even if the women does not have legal documentation to be in this country, and that she has access to resources for battered women such as medical assistance, legal advice, police assistance, and shelter.

In conclusion, the provider of services must be willing to be proactive, to serve as an advocate, to network with legal and social services, and to advocate for bilingual and bicultural services and policies. The provider must be well trained and informed to impart information about resources for legal issues, temporary restraining orders, child custody issues, and immigration issues and services.

Thus, individual services must be proactive, while respecting the woman's autonomy, self-determination, and competence. The provider needs to become an ally and a potential mentor during the early stages of treatment. Long-term support may be needed, especially if a woman decides to maintain her abusive relationship. The woman's basic worth as a human being must be respected through caring, consideration, and cultural sensitivity.

REFERENCES

Abbot J, Johnson R, Koziol-McLain J, et al: Domestic violence against women: incidence and prevalence in an emergency department population. JAMA 273:1763–1767, 1995

Amaro H, Fried LE, Cabral H, et al: Violence during pregnancy and substance abuse. Am J Public Health 80:575–579, 1990

Asbury J-E: Violence in families of color in the United States, in Family Violence: Prevention and Treatment. Edited by Hampton RL, Gullotta TP, Adams RR, et al. Newbury Park, CA, Sage, 1993, pp 159–178

Bauer HM, Rodriguez MA: Letting compassion open the door: battered women's disclosure to medical providers. Camb Q Healthc Ethics 4:459–465, 1995

Bergman B, Brismar B: A 50-year follow-up study of 117 battered women. Am J Public Health 81:1486–1489, 1991

Bograd M: Feminist perspectives on wife abuse, in Feminist Perspectives on Wife Abuse. Edited by Yllo K, Bograd M. Newbury Park, CA, Sage, 1988, pp 11–26

Brown JB, Lent B, Sas G: Identifying and treating wife abuse. J Fam Pract 36:185–191, 1993

Browne A: Violence against women by male partners, prevalence, outcomes, and policy implications. Am Psychol 48:1077–1087, 1993

Bureau of Justice Statistics: Violence Between Intimates (Publ No NCJ-149259). Washington, DC, U.S. Department of Justice, 1994

Cascardi M, Langhinrichsen J, Vivian D: Marital aggression: impact, injury and health correlates for husbands and wives. Arch Intern Med 152:1178–1184, 1992

Curtis PA: The consequences of acculturation to service delivery and research with Hispanic families. Child and Adolescent Social Work Journal 7:147–159, 1990

Dobash RE, Dobash RP: Violence Against Wives: A Case Against Patriarch. New York, Free Press, 1979

Drossman DA, Leserman J, Nachman G, et al: Sexual and physical abuse in women with functional or organic gastrointestinal disorders. Ann Intern Med 113:828–833, 1990

Ferris LE, Tudiver F: Family physician's approach to wife abuse: a study of Ontario, Canada, practices. Fam Med 24:276–282, 1992

Flores-Ortiz Y: La mujer y la violencia: a culturally based model for understanding and treatment of domestic violence in Chicana/Latina communities, in Chicana Critical Issues: Mujeres Activas en Letras y Cambio Social. Edited by Alarcon N. Berkeley, CA, Third World Women Press, 1992, pp 169–182

Flores-Ortiz Y: Fostering accountability: a reconstructive dialogue with a couple with a history of violence (Chapter 79), in 101 More Interventions in Family Therapy. Edited by Nelson T, Trepper T. New York, Haworth, 1998

Flores-Ortiz Y, Esteban M, Carrillo R: La violencia en la familia: un modelo contextual de terapia intergeneracional. Revista Interamericana de Piscologia 28:235–250, 1994

Garcia A: The changing demographic face of Hispanics in the United States, in Empowering Hispanic Families: A Critical Issue for the '90s. Edited by Sotomayor M. Milwaukee, WI, Family Service America, 1991, pp 21–38

Gin NE, Rucker L, Frayne S, et al: Prevalence of domestic violence among patients in three ambulatory care internal medicine clinics. J Gen Intern Med 6:317–322, 1991

Ginorio A, Reno J: Violence in the lives of Latina women, in The Speaking Profits Us: Violence in the Lives of Women of Color. Edited by Burns MC. Seattle, WA, Center for the Prevention of Sexual and Domestic Violence, 1986

Gondolf EW, Fisher E, McFerron JR: Racial differences among shelter residents: a comparison of Anglo, Black and Hispanic battered women. Journal of Family Violence 3:39–51, 1988

Haffner L: Translation is not enough. Interpreting in a medical setting. West J Med 157:255–259, 1992

Hamberger LK, Saunders DG, Hovey M: Prevalence of domestic violence in community practice and rate of physician inquiry. Fam Med 24:283–287, 1992

Helton AS, McFarlane J, Anderson ET: Battered and pregnant: a prevalence study. Am J Public Health 77:1337–1339, 1987

Ho CK: An analysis of domestic violence in Asian American communities: a multicultural approach to counseling. Women and Therapy (Special Issue: Diversity and Complexity in Feminist Therapy) 9(1–2):129–150, 1990

Gondolf EW, Fisher E, McFerron JR: Racial differences among shelter residents: a comparison of anglo, black, and Hispanic battered. Journal of Family Violence 3:39–51, 1988

Jalali B: Ethnicity, cultural adjustment, and behavior: implications for family therapy, in Clinical Guidelines in Cross-Cultural Mental Health. Edited by Comas-Diaz L, Griffith EEH. New York, Wiley, 1988, pp 9–32

Jang DL: Caught in a web: immigrant women and domestic violence. Clearinghouse Review 28:397–405, 1994

Kantor GK, Jasinski JL, Aldarondo E: Sociocultural status and incidence of marital violence in Hispanic families. Violence Vict 9:207–222, 1994

Koss MP, Heslet L: Somatic consequences of violence against women. Arch Fam Med 1:53–59, 1992

Kurz D: Social science perspectives on wife abuse: current debates and future directions. Gender and Society 3:489–505, 1989

Leung MT, Smith RW: Health care barriers and interventions for battered women. Public Health Reports 109:328–338, 1994

Lin MWL, Tan CI: Holding up more than half of the heavens: domestic violence in our communities, a call for justice, in The State of Asian America: Activism and Resistance in the 1990s. Edited by Aquilar-San Juan K. Boston, MA, South End Press, 1994, pp 321–333

Lockhart LL: A reexamination of the effects of race and social class on the incidence of marital violence: a search for reliable difference. Journal of Marriage and the Family 49:603–610, 1987

Marín G, Marín B: Research With Hispanic Populations. Newbury Park, CA, Sage, 1991, pp 1–41

Martinez C: Mexican Americans, in Clinical Guidelines in Cross-Cultural Mental Health. Edited by Comas-Diaz L, Griffith EEH. New York, Wiley, 1988, pp 182–201

McCauley J, Kern DE, Kolodner K: The "battering syndrome": prevalence and clinical characteristics of domestic violence in primary care internal medicine practices. Ann Intern Med 123:737–746, 1995

McFarlane J, Parker B, Soeken K, et al: Assessing for abuse during pregnancy: severity and frequency of injuries and associated entry into prenatal care. JAMA 267:3176–3178, 1992

Mirande A: The Chicano Experience: An Alternative Perspective. Notre Dame, IN, University of Notre Dame Press, 1985, pp 146–181

Mirande A, Enriquez E: La Chicana Experience: The Mexican American Woman. Chicago, IL, University of Chicago Press, 1979, pp 1–13, 96–117

Molina C, Zambrana RE, Aguirre-Molina M: The influence of culture, class, and environment on health care, in Latino Health in the United States: A Growing Challenge. Edited by Molina CW, Aguirre-Molina M. Washington, DC, American Public Health Association, 1994, pp 23–43

Neff JA, Holamon B, Schluter TD: Spousal violence among Anglos, Blacks, and Mexican Americans: the role of demographic variables, psychosocial predictors, and alcohol consumption. Journal of Family Violence 10:1–21, 1995

Panitz DR, McConchie R, Sauber SR, et al: The role of machismo and the Hispanic family in the etiology and treatment of alcoholism in Hispanic males. American Journal of Family Therapy 11:31–44, 1983

Perilla JL, Bakeman R, Norris FH: Culture and domestic violence: the ecology of abused Latinas. Violence Vict 9:325–339, 1994

Plichta S: The effects of woman abuse on health care utilization and health status: a literature review. Womens Health Issues 2:154–163, 1992

Plichta SB, Duncan MM, Plichta L: Spouse abuse, patient-physician communication and patient satisfaction. Am J Prev Med 12:297–303, 1996

Rath GD, Jarratt LG, Leonardson G: Rates of domestic violence against adult women by men partners. J Am Board Fam Pract 2:227–233, 1989

Ruiz P: Culture and mental health: a Hispanic perspective. Journal of Contemporary Psychotherapy 9:24–27, 1977

Saunders DG, Hamberger LK, Hovey M: Indicators of woman abuse based on chart review at a family practice center. Arch Fam Med 2:537–543, 1993

Sorenson SB: Violence against women: examining ethnic differences and commonalties. Evaluation Review 20:123–145, 1996

Sorenson SB, Telles CA: Self-reports of spousal violence in a Mexican American and non-Hispanic white population. Violence Vict 6:3–15, 1991

Staples R, Mirande A: Variation in family experience: racial and cultural variations among American families: a decennial review of literature on minority families, in Family in Transition: Rethinking Marriage, Sexuality, Child Rearing and Family Organization, 6th Edition. Edited by Skolnick AS, Skolnick JH. Glenview, IL, Scott, Foresman, 1989, pp 480–503

Straus MA, Smith C: Violence in Hispanic families in the United States: incidence rates and structural interpretations, in Physical Violence in American Families: Risk Factors and Adaptations to Violence in 8,145 Families. Edited by Straus MA, Gelles FR. New Brunswick, NJ, Transaction, 1989, pp 341–367

Sugg NK, Inui T: Primary care physicians' response of domestic violence: opening Pandora's box. JAMA 267:3157–3160, 1992

Torres S: A comparison of wife abuse between two cultures: perceptions, attitudes, nature and extent. Issues in Mental Health Nursing 12:113–131, 1991

Walker L: The Battered Woman. New York, Harper & Row, 1979

Warshaw C: Limitations of the medical model in the care of battered women. Gender and Society 3:506–517, 1989

Williams OJ, Becker RL: Domestic partner abuse treatment programs and cultural competence: the results of a national survey. Violence Vict 9:287–296, 1994

Woloshin S, Bickell NA, Schwartz LM, et al: Language barriers in medicine in the United States. JAMA 273:724–728, 1995

Woodward AM, Dwinell AD, Arons BS: Barriers to mental health care of Hispanic Americans: a literature review and discussion. Journal of Mental Health Administration 19:224–236, 1992

Wyatt GE: Sociocultural and epidemiological issues in the assessment of domestic violence. Journal of Social Distress and the Homeless 3:7–21, 1994

Zambrano MM: Mejor Sola que Mala Acompanada: For the Latina in an Abusive Relationship. Seattle, WA, Seal Press, 1985, pp 226–229

CHAPTER 13

Latinas in Psychiatric Treatment

Jo Ellen Brainin-Rodriguez, M.D.

IN THIS CHAPTER, I review the literature on Latina women and discuss treatment approaches that are culturally congruent. I emphasize the heterogeneous nature of the Latina population and identify critical issues to incorporate into the clinical assessment. I also cover the effect of migration, mental illness, and substance abuse on Latinas and comment on developmental gender issues. Last, I touch on resistance and feminism in the Latina community, which has become an important mental health resource.

Since the mid-1980s, a body of literature addressing the needs of female patients from both a woman-centered and a culturally competent point of view has emerged. Popular mainstream psychological literature is beginning to reflect this accumulated body of knowledge (Gil and Vazquez 1996). The influx of women of color into women's studies centers of academic institutions and the development of a feminist developmental perspective in psychology have created a body of literature that integrates clinical practice with feminist analysis and a cross-cultural perspective (Amaro and Russo 1987).

To understand Latinas in context requires a clear understanding of their social conditions, their individual circumstances, and the relationships that govern their cultural milieu, including class, age, race, and gender issues. The specific conditions that lead to a Latina's migration; the source of her social support; her views about marriage and gender equality; and her perception of her social options all affect a woman's world view and ultimately her mental health (Arguelles and

Rivero 1995; Espin 1987; Zayas and Busch-Rossnagel 1992).

Latinas are not a monolithic group. The demographic characteristics and psychosocial stressors vary greatly among the different groups. Therefore, it is important to examine gender roles within the context of the majority culture as well as within the cultural milieu of the woman. For example, race/ethnicity and sexual preference may set a woman apart within the Latino culture of origin, exposing her to greater stress and fewer options. A black Cuban woman, a woman of Mesquito Indian ancestry from Nicaragua, and a Puerto Rican lesbian may have clinical issues that differ from those of the mainstream of each of these countries. Social policy and treatment options will be more comprehensive and more likely to be effective if a multidimensional view of Latinas is applied in assessment.

MIGRATION

For Latinas who have migrated, the migration experience is often a pivotal event in their lives. Migration can bring expanded opportunities in the areas of education and employment, but the new social environment can present conflicts of roles and values. These conflicts can negatively affect mental health, causing anxiety and depression (Bernal and Gutierrez 1988; Martinez 1988; Ramos-McKay et al. 1988). Latinas who are at highest risk for psychological problems as a result of poor adjustment to the migration experience are those who have migrated involuntarily, who have lost their protective caregivers and other support systems, and who have had a decline in social and economic status (Espin 1987).

Migration may have several antecedents. Although often it is propelled by economic need, other factors must be considered. For example, the role of migration in Puerto Rican culture may be a response to interpersonal stresses such as divorce, illness, or conflict of cross-generational values. Parents often send a teenager from the island to New York or vice versa to deal with an adolescent crisis. Precipitants may be a romantic relationship that the parents disapprove of, trouble with school, or trouble with the law. Economic difficulties may cause a parent to send children to live with grandparents or other relatives. Although this may relieve the situation in the short run, the children or adolescents may be left without important supports and may have to cope with numerous new stresses as a result of the move (Bernal and Flores-Ortiz 1982). If migration follows major traumatic events, such as parental loss, sexual assault, or war, the move and need to adapt to a new social milieu and language may prove to be too overwhelming for a healthy accommodation.

Arguelles and Rivero (1995) emphasized that when assessing Latina immigrants or refugees, gender-specific factors leading to migration must be considered, such as gender violence, enforced gender roles, sexual orientation, sexual abuse and assault, and coerced motherhood. Central American women's migration may be precipitated by traumatic events such as loss of a parent, sexual assault, or family conflict (Vargas-Willis and Cervantes 1987). The following case example illustrates some of these issues:

> Ms. N, a 19-year-old undocumented Salvadoran woman who migrated to the United States with a male cousin, was hospitalized for intense suicidal ideation and auditory hallucinations that emerged over a few days. She had left El Salvador after she had been kidnapped and brutally raped by soldiers of the National Guard. In the 4 months since Ms. N arrived in the United States, she had been working as a housekeeper in a hotel, despite having nightmares and anxiety. Most recently, she had started dating a young man who was pressuring her for a sexual relationship. She left her cousin's home because "there were a lot of guys there," and she felt threatened by them. Her housing situation was precarious because she was staying with a female co-worker on a temporary basis.

This case illustrates how socioeconomic stresses, loss of familial support, and prior unresolved traumatic experiences conspire to create a situation in which even a resourceful and independent young woman was too overwhelmed to continue to function. For women who are undocumented, the vulnerability they experience in situations of exploitation such as domestic violence or sexual harassment at work can be the source of tremendous stress and contribute to many psychiatric symptoms. In the case of Ms. N, the loss of family support, the triggers of the sexualized relationship, and the housing situation in which she perceived herself to be at risk for sexual assault were the conditions that tipped the scales of her precarious adjustment.

Interventions focused on reestablishing social supports. Ms. N was referred to a Spanish-speaking counselor at a rape treatment center, who not only assisted with treatment of the trauma but also helped her find a safe housing situation. Her female co-worker emerged as a support, who allowed Ms. N to stay at her place until she was able to find a room in the house of a family where she did not feel sexually threatened. Her auditory hallucinations and suicidal ideation resolved after administration of a low-dose antipsychotic; when the physician discontinued the medication a week later, the symptoms did not recur.

The diagnoses were severe posttraumatic stress disorder (PTSD), with brief reactive psychosis and depressed mood. The interventions helped her repair ruptured social bonds, which Herman (1993) described as the central effect of severe trauma. In Ms. N's case, the political nature of the sexual assault made her a candidate for working with church-based agencies familiar with the social circumstances of refugees from Central America. It was also important to acknowledge the stress of her undocumented legal status and to refer her to agencies that could assist her. The involuntary hospitalization also exacerbated the feeling of loss of control over her life and the fear that she would be turned over to immigration authorities, so efforts were made to reassure her and to allow as much control as possible over the conditions in the hospital.

MENTAL ILLNESS AND SUBSTANCE ABUSE

Clinical evidence suggests that women with mental illness or substance abuse are more likely to be abandoned by their partners than are men with similar problems (Beckman and Amaro 1986; Lex 1991). In Latino families, the stigma of mental illness and substance abuse is often increased for women because of their inability to meet expectations such as primary caregiving of children and nurturing the rest of the family. Latinas are therefore at risk for losing an important source of support, as well as an important source of self-esteem in fulfilling expected roles in the family.

Latina patterns of alcohol use have been studied in Mexicans, Puerto Ricans, and Cubans. The trends described in the 1984 Hispanic Health and Nutrition Examination Survey (HHANES) data indicated that Latina women drink less than men do and that traditional sanctions against women drinking appear to exist (Aguirre-Molina and Caetano 1994). However, according to more recent studies, acculturation and education appear to weaken the injunctions against drinking in Latinas. Female single heads of household appear to drink more than married females. Flores-Ortiz (1994) found that Latinas attending high school and college have considerable difficulty moderating alcohol consumption in the context of courting and sexual situations and that in spite of knowledge, information, and high levels of perceived self-efficacy, few actually have changed high-risk behaviors. For example, few young women understood that alcohol consumption increased their risk of sexually transmitted diseases, including human immunodeficiency virus (HIV).

The following case example illustrates issues common to Latinas who are dependent on alcohol or drugs.

Ms. O, a 32-year-old Puerto Rican woman, was arrested for soliciting sex and later transferred to a locked medical ward for treatment of a kidney infection. The psychiatric consultation service was called in to evaluate her because she was experiencing intense suicidal ideation.

Ms. O, who was bilingual but more comfortable speaking English, reported recent heroin use and a 1-year history of intravenous drug addiction.

Her drug use led to her losing custody of her daughters, ages 4 and 6 years. They were placed in the custody of Ms. O's mother. The daughters' father was in prison and also abused drugs. Before his imprisonment, the domestic situation had been violent.

On psychiatric assessment, Ms. O was found to be overwhelmed with shame, helplessness, hopelessness, and extreme anxiety. She was having fantasies of throwing herself through a window but observed that the windows in the medical ward were "too small." Her worries included fear that she would never regain custody of her daughters. In the course of the evaluation, she reported that her girls were "all I live for" and proudly displayed pictures of them. She had an appointment with the jail social worker, who was helping her get into a drug rehabilitation program. To gain acceptance, she was expected to write a letter stating her goals but reported feeling too overwhelmed to do so. She was also a heavy smoker and having a "nicotine fit" and bargaining to let her "have a smoke."

The immediate intervention consisted of helping her prioritize her worries to decrease her anxiety. To regain custody of her children, she needed to participate in drug treatment, so the task of writing her goals letter was primary. Because she had identified her daughters as the reason to "keep going," the Latina consultant helped her make a small bedside altar with the photographs of the daughters and a vase of flowers. She then began writing the letter, with the pictures of the girls serving as her inspiration. Her craving for cigarettes could only be accommodated with nicotine gum. This was reframed for her as a "test" of what she was going to experience when she entered recovery. Thinking about her daughters also gave her the needed courage to overcome her craving. When speaking about the girls, the doctor often made statements such as *"Que bonitas, Dios las guarde"* (How pretty they are, God bless them). The compliment framed a protective blessing, acknowledging Ms. O's desire to be a protector of her children and in keeping with the Puerto Rican custom to bless children after admiring them to protect them from *mal de ojo* (evil eye). The bilingualism of both the patient and the provider allowed the doctor to switch from English to Spanish to emphasize particular topics, to give these topics different emotional valence, and to facilitate discussion of taboo issues (Espin 1987). The recommendations to the medical team included monitoring of signs of physiological withdrawal and brief, reassuring contacts with Ms. O during the day.

DEVELOPMENTAL GENDER ISSUES

Latinas contend with stereotypes related to gender both outside and within their own culture. The view outside the culture of Latinas as passive, ultrafeminine, and not particularly intelligent or ambitious may inhibit their aspirations and educational opportunities. Similarly, the Latina may be inhibited from reaching her potential within the patriarchal family structure that sees achievement as a masculine trait and encourages females to relegate themselves to activities within the home and family.

The experience of adolescence is often one of turmoil and transition. The values of one's family of origin are often called into question and identity is in flux as an adolescent struggles with a myriad of developmental tasks, such as sexual identity and desire, role demands in the family, and peer pressures to conform. Young people in the United States, regardless of cultural background, are more likely to have much unsupervised time and to be coping with a peer culture that is in opposition to the values of their culture of origin. This may cause a difficult situation for Latina adolescents as they cope with pressures to enter into early sexual relationships and simultaneously lose the protection of the traditional family structure that keeps young women well chaperoned. A conflict exists between the traditional values of the "cult of virginity" and men as seducers and the permissive values of contemporary American sexual mores. This increases the likelihood that young women will engage in early sexual activity as the peer injunctions lessen and familial supervision diminishes. The risks for young Latinas engaging in early sexual activity include ostracism from relatives for dishonoring the family name once she is not a virgin, sexually transmitted diseases, teen pregnancy, and the emotional stress of sexually intensified romantic pairings and partings.

During adolescence, many Latinas may reject traditional gender roles in their family. This may create conflict for them if they are no longer willing to fulfill the role of dutiful daughter as an extension of the mother in the home (e.g., baby-sitting younger siblings or attending to household chores after school).

In families undergoing cross-generational conflicts, the alienation between mother and daughter may cost the young Latina one of her strongest advocates in coming to terms with the stresses of the majority culture. For Latinas, questioning patriarchal values within and outside the culture brings them face to face with a devalued self-concept. For their mothers, the conflict may be experienced as one of traditional values being rejected by their daughters, even when they themselves struggle in the workplace or in a marriage against similar issues. The unacknowledged desire to help their daughters fit into the prescribed molds may be motivated by wanting to spare their daughters the pain of being different or at odds with cultural norms but may leave young girls feeling alone and alienated from potential sources of support.

Studies examining the self-concept of preadolescent girls documented a dramatic decline in self-concept and self-confidence, especially between grade school and junior high school. This decline in self-concept leads to an inhibition of actions and abilities (Debold et al. 1994). Although these data are not exclusively about Latinas, the *familismo* (family interdependence and loyalty) of the Latino culture may suggest a way of greater protection that can be provided for girls' healthy development within the structure of the family. Debold's concept of "the family as safe house" has much to offer. Family-focused therapy with Latino families engages them in the task of providing an environment for their daughters that is actively antisexist.

The following case example illustrates the effects of invoking a father's protective role vis-à-vis his daughter to encourage substance abuse treatment.

> Mr. and Mrs. P, a middle-aged Latino couple, sought treatment because of Mr. P's alcoholism and verbal abuse toward his wife. Mr. P was quite defensive in the assessment, minimizing the effects of his behavior on the family. He repeatedly stated, "At least I don't hit her anymore," and he minimized his drinking problem. During the treatment course, the therapist pointed out that because the couple's adolescent daughter was witnessing these episodes of verbal abuse, she might come to believe that this is the way women are treated in relationships. The therapist then asked Mr. P, "Is this what you want for her?" He became very quiet and answered, "Yes, I guess that it is true," and for the first time accepted a referral to a Latino-focused alcohol treatment agency.

The father's realization of the effect that his behavior had in shaping his daughter's perception of how husband-and-wife relationships were, and his desire to ensure her safety in future relationships, decreased his resistance to treatment.

LATINA WOMEN IN THE LATER YEARS

Aging Latinas as a group are poorer than their white counterparts and can be considered, like other aging minority women, to embody the "quadruple jeopardy" of being old, poor, female, and of minority status. Approximately 50% of elderly Latinas live in poverty compared with 20% of all elderly women. The research that examines the role of ethnicity, socioeconomic status, gender, and age is conflicted regarding the exact meaning of their interaction, but it appears that—particularly in the group of women older than 85—low income is not necessarily linked to lower levels of social support, family interaction, and self-reported life satisfaction or high mortality. There appears to be some support for the notion of adaptive successful aging among some minority women. The strategies that help them survive to old age pay off in increased resourcefulness and self-reliance (Padgett 1989).

As Latinas age, they are more likely to be involved in the lives of their children (e.g., cooking, giving advice, and performing other emotionally supportive tasks). The social status of many Latinas increases as they age and elicit the *respeto* (respect) from their children and grandchildren around them. The reciprocity inherent in the value of *familismo* may be expressed in the exchange of a supportive role in the family of their children and the economic support of the children with assistance during times of ill health. The presence of a mental disorder in an aging Latina, along with the economic difficulties of urban life in the United States, can stress these transgenerational expectations.

The following case example illustrates the effect of economic reality on the extended family structure.

> Mrs. Q, a 64-year-old Mexican-born mother of three adult children, was admitted to the inpatient psychiatric service in an acute manic crisis. Although she had been given the diagnosis of bipolar affective disorder many years ago, she had been relatively stable until in recent years, when her episodes of mania became more frequent. A traditional church-attending woman, Mrs. Q baby-sat her grandchildren and cooked their meals while their parents worked. She was brought to the hospital by her husband and eldest daughter, who were worried because she "couldn't take care of things anymore." They reported that she had become increasingly irritable, doing little more at home than praying loudly, and that she had become erotically preoccupied with the priest in their parish. During previous hospitalizations, Mr. Q had avoided family meetings, stating over the telephone, "just tell me when I can come pick her up."

The adult children and their spouses had to work outside the home; thus, the family system had less flexibility to weather the incapacity of the elder caretaker of the children. For Mr. Q, the stigma of his wife's illness contributed to his avoidance of the treatment team, so he did not have education about his wife's illness and treatment options. Interventions in this type of case would include not only psychopharmacology and milieu treatment but also aggressive efforts to involve the extended family in the treatment. If the family is not knowledgeable and supportive of the treatment plan, the urgency of their own need for Mrs. Q to resume her duties may undermine the rehabilitation by returning her too soon to the usual family responsibilities.

Many traditional family responses may not be available in the setting of the United States when confronted with the needs of aging Latinas. Overcrowding may interfere with the family's taking in of aging mothers who can no longer live independently. The acculturation of grandchildren may decrease the status of grandparenting, and grandchildren may see their grandparents as old-fashioned. They may have difficulty communicating because the grandchildren do not speak Spanish. Women who migrate later in life also may be particularly isolated by the lack of language skills, increased risk of street crime, or loss of community supports in the country of origin.

FEMINISM IN THE LATINO COMMUNITY

Stereotypes of Latinas often portray a submissive woman who is dominated first by her father and later by her spouse and who is mistreated in her relationships. An examination of social reality speaks a different story. It is important to appreciate that within each culture are numerous subcultures. In Latino culture, as in perhaps most cultures, the sociopolitical reality of women and men is quite different. In cultures in which women are oppressed by social institutions, a "culture of resistance" exists that, to a greater or lesser extent, functions in a parallel fashion. For example, coalitions of women involved in efforts to combat economic inequality and violence against women exist in every Latin American country. As an example, in the *Directorio de ONG de Nicaragua 1993–1995* [*Directory of Non-Governmental Organizations of Nicaragua 1993–1995*], of the 160 organizations listed, at least 20 identify their primary purpose to be the promotion of gender equality and women's rights (Littlejohn 1993). Similar observations can be made internationally, as evidenced by the platform of the Beijing Women's Conference (Pietila and Vickers 1994). The subsuming of women's oppression as "part of the culture" is not a point of view endorsed by Latina women as a whole.

From the United States perspective, female resistance to domestic violence, inequities in the legal rights of women in marriage, and other social ills that affect women differentially are not the exclusive province of the American feminist movement. Many Latinas who emigrate from impoverished areas of Latin America may have been exposed to labor organizations or other venues where they have struggled to assert themselves despite social resistance to their demands. Furthermore, across Latin America and the Caribbean, a lively debate and social movement for women's rights have been very present, encouraged by Leftist movements, especially the Cuban and later Nicaraguan revolutions (Vukelich and Gist 1996).

This sensibility is reflected in many of the indigenous support networks that can be seen in the urban centers of the United States, where many Latinas live (Young and Padilla 1990). For example, in San Francisco, California, Mujeres Unidas y Activas is an organization that supports Latina immigrants who are exploited in domestic work. Services provided include discussions on numerous topics of interest to Latinas, such as orientations to health and legal services as well as support groups for women in abusive relationships.

The following case example illustrates the effects of involvement with Latina support groups.

Ms. R, a young Mexican woman, used the support of a Latina women's organization to get a restraining order against her physically abusive husband. The support group she participated in encouraged her to demand that he follow through with treatment in a group for battering men. After he did, they were reunited, and she continued involvement with the group by providing advocacy for other women who needed to interface with the legal system.

Ms. R described herself as *muy cambiada* (very changed) as a result of her contact with the group. She became outgoing and took pride in her contribution to the community. In the course of her work, she even spoke to a class of 130 medical students who were studying the cultural aspects of domestic violence about her personal experiences.

TREATMENT ISSUES AND STRATEGIES

Particular characteristics in a therapist or provider enhance rapport and engagement with the Latina patient in the clinical setting. Although these issues may be less important in the acculturated patient, it is wise to consider them early on in the treatment, especially if the therapist has some difficulties in engaging with the patient.

If the primary or dominant language of a patient is Spanish, then it is important for the assessment and treatment to be provided in Spanish. Patients who may be quite psychotic often use English to mask the extent of their symptoms. For example, a bilingual woman who was evaluated in English expressed suicidal ideation, but when the interview was switched to Spanish, she revealed elaborate paranoid delusions, and the severity of the suicidal ideation became more prominent. In another case, an elderly woman with rudimentary knowledge of English was interviewed in English and found to be "somewhat concrete, raising the possibility of mild dementia." When she was reinterviewed in Spanish, a full affect and intellectual capacity were evident.

Because of the cultural value of *machismo*, which among other elements describes males as preoccupied with sexual conquest and domination over other males who threaten the family, Latinas may have difficulty trusting male providers with very personal issues, especially those related to marital conflict and sexuality. However, if rapport is established, a male provider, especially a Latino, can be well positioned to model for Latino families that being male does not require subordination of others. Male therapists must be attentive to when the gender difference interferes with the Latina patient's openness and must maintain a demeanor that is sufficiently formal so that it cannot be interpreted as flirting or sexualized behavior.

CONCLUSIONS

In summary, when addressing issues of psychiatric treatment, the provider must be aware of the diversity of the Latina population and his or her own particular biases and perspectives. Recent immigration status, poverty, or lack of formal education does not automatically mean that a woman accepts a patriarchal belief system. An attitude of respectful inquiry about a particular woman's experience and psychosocial reality, including support system, immigration history (if relevant), and experience with gender and racial discrimination, should be part of any psychiatric evaluation. It is especially important to be aware of heterosexist bias because lesbians of color are a particularly invisible minority. Experiences of discrimination may occur both within and outside the culture, as, for example, experienced by Latinas of indigenous or African descent.

In clinical work with Latinas, it is often helpful to analyze the patient's situation from the point of view of multiple role conflicts and to reframe the difficulties from that perspective. Attention should be paid to ensure that the assessment and interventions are conducted in the language the patient is most fluent and comfortable in. It is also important that family and other supports be involved in treatment planning. Enhanced knowledge of cross-cultural issues in the psychological care of Latinas is an area in rich evolution at present. As the largest growing minority group in the United States, Latinas are bound to be part of the clinical practice of clinicians everywhere.

REFERENCES

Aguirre-Molina M, Caetano R: Alcohol use and alcohol-related issues, in Latino Health in the US: A Growing Challenge. Edited by Molina CW, Aguirre-Molina M. Washington, DC, American Public Health Association, 1994, pp 400–401

Amaro H, Russo NF: Hispanic women and mental health: an overview of contemporary issues in research and practice. Psychology of Women Quarterly 11:393–407, 1987

Arguelles L, Rivero A: Violence, migration and compassionate practice: conversations with some Latinas we think we know, in Racism in the Lives of Women: Testimony, Theory and Guides to Antiracist Practice. Edited by Adleman J, Enguidanos G. New York, Harrington Park Press, 1995, pp 149–160

Beckman L, Amaro H: Personal and social difficulties faced by women and men entering alcoholism treatment. J Stud Alcohol 47:135–145, 1986

Bernal G, Flores-Ortiz Y: Latino families in therapy: engagement and evaluation. Journal of Marital and Family Therapy 8:357–365, 1982

Bernal G, Gutierrez M: Cubans, in Clinical Guidelines in Cross-Cultural Mental Health. Edited by Comas-Diaz L, Griffith EEH. New York, Wiley, 1988, pp 233–261

Debold E, Wilson M, Malave I: Mother Daughter Revolution: From Good Girls to Great Women. New York, Bantam Books, 1994

Espin O: Psychological impact of migration on Latinas: implications for psychotherapeutic practice. Psychology of Women Quarterly 11:489–503, 1987

Flores-Ortiz Y: The role of cultural and gender values in alcohol use patterns among Chicana/Latina high school and university students: implications for AIDS prevention. Int J Addict 29:1149–1171, 1994

Gil RM, Vazquez CI: The Maria Paradox: How Latinas Can Merge Old World Traditions With New World Self-Esteem. New York, GP Putnam's Sons, 1996

Herman J: Trauma and Recovery. New York, Basic Books, 1993

Lex BW: Some gender differences in alcohol and polysubstance users. Health Psychol 10:121–132, 1991

Littlejohn C: Directorio de ONG de Nicaragua 1993–1995. Managua, Nicaragua, Centro de Apoyo a Programas y Proyectos (CAPRI), 1993

Martinez C: Mexican Americans, in Clinical Guidelines in Cross-Cultural Mental Health. Edited by Comas-Diaz L, Griffith EEH. New York, Wiley, 1988, pp 182–203

Padgett D: Aging minority women: issues in research and health policy, in Women in the Later Years: Health, Social and Cultural Perspectives. Edited by Grau L, Susser I. New York, Harrington Park Press, 1989, pp 173–181

Pietila H, Vickers J: Making Women Matter: The Role in the United Nations. Atlantic Highlands, NJ, Zed Books, 1994

Ramos-McKay JM, Comas-Diaz L, Rivera LA: Puerto Ricans, in Clinical Guidelines in Cross-Cultural Mental Health. Edited by Comas-Diaz L, Griffith EEH. New York, Wiley, 1988, pp 204–232

Vargas-Willis C, Cervantes RC: Considerations of psychosocial stress in the treatment of the Latina immigrant. Hispanic Journal of Behavioral Sciences 9:315–329, 1987

Vukelich D, Gist D: The Council of Evangelical Churches of Nicaragua. Eagle Creek, OR, Alton L Collins Retreat Center, 1996

Young E, Padilla M: Mujeres unidas en accion: a popular education process. Community Based Education 2 (60; Special Issue):1–18, 1990

Zayas LH, Busch-Rossnagel NH: Pregnant Hispanic women: a mental health study: families in society. Journal of Contemporary Human Services 73(9):515–521, 1992

CHAPTER 14

Substance Abuse in the Hispanic Population

Louis R. Alvarez, M.D., M.P.H.

SUBSTANCE ABUSE IS CONSIDERED by many to be the number one public health problem in the United States (Botvin et al. 1995). More deaths, illnesses, and disabilities are caused by substance abuse than by any other preventable health condition (Schneider Institute for Health Policy, Brandeis University 1993). Significant segments of the Hispanic American population have been devastated by alcohol and drug abuse (Soriano 1994). Hispanics are among the most severely affected of all groups because of unique sociocultural conditions. For many Hispanics, drugs and alcohol are major social anesthetics from the pain of poverty, discrimination, and underemployment. The increasingly conservative tenor of the times, reduced access to health care, inadequate health insurance coverage, and disproportionately less federal spending on treatment than on law enforcement are fueling the substance abuse crisis among Hispanics (Greig 1996). The Hispanic population will more than triple in size from 24 million in 1992 to a projected 81 million in 2050 (U.S. Bureau of the Census 1992). Because this population is growing at such an accelerated pace, the effect of substance abuse will be catastrophically magnified as more Hispanics are affected.

This chapter is meant to serve as a practical guide for health care professionals working with Hispanic patients with the pernicious problem of substance abuse. It seeks to advance an understanding of the sociocultural and demographic variables that are important when evaluating and treating substance abuse in Hispanics. Although certain cultural values, attitudes, and norms are shared by many Hispanic subgroups, one of this chapter's central tenets is that treatment providers should not assume that one approach will work for all Hispanics. The values pertaining to the Hispanic person's particular subgroup significantly influence drug-using patterns and affect how substance abuse is manifested. Because of the labyrinthine nature of substance abuse, treatment programs must offer strategies that are comprehensive and targeted to the specific Hispanic subgroups they serve. In this chapter, I provide an overview of approaches that have been effective in the treatment of drug-abusing Hispanics. This chapter does not pretend to be an exhaustive review of all the available treatment modalities. I focus on the 1) epidemiology of substance abuse in Hispanics, 2) etiology of substance abuse in Hispanics, 3) cultural issues in the treatment of substance abuse in Hispanics, and 4) principles of treatment of substance abuse in Hispanics.

EPIDEMIOLOGY OF SUBSTANCE ABUSE

Although it is not within the scope of this chapter to discuss at great length the epidemiology of substance abuse among Hispanic Americans, it must be understood that drug use patterns vary by Hispanic subgroup, age group, and region of the United States. Research has found that substance use among Hispanics is generally lower than that among white non-Hispanic individuals, although Hispanic use may be higher for some substances (cocaine, crack cocaine, heroin) (Chavez and Swaim 1992). The variations in much of the literature may be due in large part to the cultural diversity and inherent complexity of the Hispanic population (Chavez and Swaim 1992). The reader is referred elsewhere (National Institute on Drug Abuse 1995; Ruiz and Langrod 1997) for a detailed epidemiology of the specific drugs used by various Hispanic subgroups.

The principal difficulty with studies of substance use among Hispanic subgroups has been the inability to obtain adequate sample sizes to achieve reliable estimates of use among these subgroups. It is essential to recognize that the various subgroups that compose the Hispanic population in the United States are demographically different, with distinct cultural traditions and histories and unique immigration and assimilation experiences. These differences are likely to account for some of the disparities in substance use among these subgroups (Chavez 1993).

The following studies provide evidence of the gravity of the drug problem in the Hispanic population. Research (National Health Interview Survey

1992) on the prevalence of drug use among Hispanics indicates that it is alarmingly high among youth. Because a large proportion of the Hispanic population is young—median Hispanic age in the United States is 25.3 years compared with 32.8 years for the overall United States population—a larger proportion of Hispanics may be at increased risk for drug use (U.S. Bureau of the Census 1992). In the 12- to 15-year age group, Hispanic boys reported the highest lifetime and past-month uses of alcohol, marijuana, cocaine, and crack cocaine when compared with whites and African Americans (National Health Interview Survey 1992). A 1994 Monitoring the Future Study (National Institute on Drug Abuse 1994) reported that Hispanics in the eighth grade had the highest rates of use for most drugs, including tobacco, compared with white and African American populations. Among eighth graders, 23.3% of the Hispanic students reported ever having used marijuana, compared with 13.2% of the African American students and 12.9% of the white students (National Institute on Drug Abuse 1994). Hispanic eighth graders had the highest rate of binge drinking (22.3%), compared with 12.9% for whites and 11.8% for African Americans (National Institute on Drug Abuse 1994). Hispanic students in the 1993 Youth Risk Behavior Surveillance System Survey (Centers for Disease Control and Prevention 1995) were more than twice as likely to have used cocaine in their lifetime (11.3%), compared with white and African American students (4.4% and 1.6%, respectively). Lifetime use of crack cocaine or freebase forms of cocaine was highest among Hispanic students (6.3%), followed by white and African American students (2.3 and 1.1%, respectively) (Centers for Disease Control and Prevention 1995). This is quite unsettling because, of the various forms of cocaine, the smokable form (crack or freebase) has the greatest addictive potential (Gold 1992).

The heavy substance use among youth is troubling because the data (Huba et al. 1981) indicate that, among adolescents, the earlier in life drug use begins, the more likely that drug use will increase with each subsequent year. Because adolescents are undergoing momentous changes, including identity development and the learning of adaptive coping responses, an interruption in these processes by drug use has lifelong consequences (Felix-Ortiz et al. 1994). Research (Felix-Ortiz et al. 1994) indicates that Hispanic adolescents may be at special risk for drug use because of emotional distress. The high level of poverty and low level of educational attainment place Hispanic youth at higher risk for emotional distress compared with the general United States population. The profound degree of emotional distress and deep despair experienced by Hispanic youth is tragically reflected in reports (Youth Risk Behavior Survey Data 1991) that Hispanic adolescents were most likely to have attempted suicide. Data from the 1991 Youth Risk Behavior Survey showed that 12.0% of the Hispanic high school students reported attempting suicide at least once compared with 7.9% of the white students and 6.5% of the African American students.

Alcohol and other drug use has been found to be a high predictor of attempted suicide among Puerto Ricans (Fernandez-Pol et al. 1986). The higher rates of drug use among Puerto Ricans may partially explain their higher rates of suicide (J. Ungemack and P. Guarnaccia, "Suicidal Ideation and Suicide Attempts Among Hispanics in the United States," unpublished manuscript, New Brunswick, NJ, Rutgers University Institute of Health, Health Care Policy, and Aging, 1993). An important point is that the current estimates of drug use in Hispanic youth, although disproportionately high, probably grossly underestimate the true extent of the problem because Hispanics have the highest school dropout rates, making reliable estimates difficult to obtain (Johnston et al. 1991). In addition, studies (Mensch and Kandel 1988) found that Hispanic and African American youth were more likely than white youth to underreport their use of drugs. It is believed that because of strong cultural sanctions against drug use by women, the degree of underreporting by Hispanic women is undetermined. The double standard among Hispanics, which minimizes the male's use of drugs but is very censorious of the female's use, is an especially powerful contributor to surreptitious alcohol use by Hispanic women (Caetano 1988). Most of the literature (Substance Abuse and Mental Health Services Administration 1993), however, has reported that Hispanic women are less likely than white women to use alcohol, tobacco, and other drugs.

Among the more troubling findings in drug use studies are data (Maddahian et al. 1985) that show that Hispanics are the group most frequently engaged in the use of multiple drugs compared with other populations. Most disturbing are data from 1993 Drug Abuse Warning Network (DAWN) survey (Substance Abuse and Mental Health Services Administration 1994), which indicated that Hispanics have the highest percentage of accidental drug-related deaths (80.5%), compared with African Americans (62.9%) and whites (51.8%). In 1993, heroin or morphine was reported in 61% of the cases when the decedent in a drug-related death was Hispanic, 45% when the decedent was African American, and 41% when the decedent was white (U.S. Department of Health and Human Services et al. 1993). Also appalling are DAWN data from a 1988–1993 survey (Substance Abuse and Mental Health Services Administration 1994) of drug-related emergency room visits for those aged 12–17, showing a decrease for whites (6%) and African Americans (14%) but an increase of 36% for Hispanics in the same age group. In emergency room drug-related episodes for Hispanics, cocaine was involved in 25.6% and heroin or morphine in 23.4% of the episodes (Substance Abuse and Mental Health Services Administration 1994). Drug-related deaths and emergency room visits are the two most serious indicators of problematic drug use and serve as barometers of the severity of drug-related health complications. They clearly show the enormity of the substance abuse problem among Hispanics in communities where drug use is rampant. It is not unreasonable to postulate that higher rates of multiple drug use and/or greater quantities of drugs ingested among Hispanics may be key factors in their greater number of drug-related emergency room visits and accidental deaths (Oetting and Beauvais 1990).

An in-depth discussion of the various substances of abuse used by Hispanics is beyond the scope of this chapter, and the reader is referred elsewhere (National Institute on Drug Abuse 1995; Ruiz and Langrod 1997). It is worthwhile, nonetheless, to highlight some key points of certain drugs that have particular relevance for clinicians working with the Hispanic population. Research (Gilbert 1985) suggests that Hispanics are at greater risk for alcohol abuse because alcohol is woven into the social fabric of family and community life, and its traditional convivial use is well accepted. To a significant extent, drinking is also accepted for its utilitarian use as a method of reducing stress and anxiety. Studies (Caetano 1984) have found that Hispanics have more liberal attitudes toward alcohol use and intoxication than do African Americans and whites, which may help to explain the higher rates of use and alcohol-related problems among Hispanics. Existing data sources (Aguirre-Molina and Caetano 1994) unambiguously indicate that alcohol-related diseases strike Hispanics disproportionately and that Hispanics are overrepresented among alcohol-related deaths. Data from the National Center for Health Statistics (1990) ranked chronic liver disease and cirrhosis as the sixth and seventh most frequent causes of death in Puerto Ricans and Mexican Americans, respectively, whereas they ranked tenth among whites and African Americans. The increased use of marijuana among certain Hispanic populations is also of concern because, like alcohol, it is a gateway drug and often leads to other drug use (Kandel and Yamaguchi 1993). Research (A. Leshner, Director, NIDA, statement at the press conference for the release of the 1994 Monitoring the Future Survey, December 12, 1994) demonstrates that cognition may be affected to the point of hampering the acquisition of new knowledge when students use marijuana. The implications of this finding are dire when one considers that this deleterious effect on learning may further increase the already vast numbers of Hispanics dropping out of school.

Although general population studies have not found that Hispanics are more likely than non-Hispanic whites to use inhalants, there appear to be circumscribed areas, such as the United States–Mexico border region, where there are silent epidemics of inhalant abuse (Mata and Rodriguez-Andrew

1988). Several studies (Rouse 1986) indicate that Hispanics use inhalants earlier because of easy access, with reports of use in children as young as 7 years. Because many antidrug campaigns have tended to ignore inhalants, many Hispanic youth are unaware that they can be as lethal as cocaine or heroin and cause irreversible brain, kidney, and liver damage following chronic exposure. Most experts feel that fatalities are underreported, especially among the typical Hispanic users who are impoverished "street children" from broken homes. A serious concern related to those Hispanics who abuse inhalants is that, like alcohol and marijuana, inhalants are a gateway drug and often part of a poly-drug pattern of drug use.

Perhaps nowhere else has the effect of substance abuse on the Hispanic American population been more devastating than in the transmission of the human immunodeficiency virus (HIV). Although Hispanics constitute only 10% of the United States population, the Centers for Disease Control and Prevention (1996) reported that through December 1996, Hispanics accounted for 19% of the cumulative acquired immunodeficiency syndrome (AIDS) cases, or almost twice their United States representation. It is a telling index of the egregious effect of Hispanic injection drug use on HIV transmission that, of these cumulative AIDS cases, 37% of the Hispanic males (compared with 9% of the non-Hispanic white males) and 44% of the Hispanic females contracted HIV through injection drug use (Centers for Disease Control and Prevention 1996). Among the cumulative number of Hispanic pediatric AIDS cases reported through December 1996, an alarming 63% were attributable to the mother's engaging in injection drug use or having sex with an injection drug user.

ETIOLOGY OF SUBSTANCE ABUSE

Drug use among Hispanic Americans is a complex and multidetermined behavior. The literature (Ruiz and Langrod 1997) that exists on this subject suggests that significant factors in the etiology of addiction among Hispanics are socioculturally related to a considerable extent. Although an in-depth discussion of economic and social policy lies outside the purview of this chapter, it must be emphasized that they are of paramount importance in any attempt to discern the etiology of substance abuse in the Hispanic population.

In analyzing the various conditions that predispose Hispanics to substance abuse, it is undeniably clear that poverty is the single greatest risk factor. Family poverty is inextricably linked to high rates of drug use and academic failure. The condition of poverty immeasurably intensifies the suffering and adversity experienced by the Hispanic substance abuser by amplifying the virulent social and health-related consequences of drug use. Hispanics are manifestly overrepresented among the poor (Sue and Sue 1990). Since 1987, the poverty rate has declined significantly for African Americans and whites, whereas the Hispanic rate has increased (Porter et al. 1988). According to the U.S. Bureau of the Census (1995), the proportion of Hispanics living in poverty has risen from 21.9% in 1973 to 30.3% in 1995. Research (Kail 1993) has indicated that socioeconomic status may be more highly related to drug abuse among Hispanics than among African Americans and whites. Poverty may be a crucial factor in prompting high rates of drug use among Hispanics because it provides few life choices and resources to buffer the inordinate stress and strain experienced by the Hispanic family of low socioeconomic status. The creators of the woefully inadequate "Just Say No" campaign against drug use regrettably failed to realize that society has not given impecunious and marginalized minorities enough to say yes to. Economic hardship has left many Hispanics devoid of hope for a better life and with little capacity to cope. This has promoted an attitude of "living for the moment," which is a significant disincentive to reducing drug use. Hispanic youth are exceedingly vulnerable to negative influences and peer pressure to experiment with drugs when they experience inequality, discrimination, and economic insecurity in United States society. The literature (Booth et al. 1990) consistently reports among Hispanic youth that a friend's use of a drug is the greatest single factor influencing initiation and continuation of drug use.

The strong relation between dropping out of school and the use of drugs has been well documented by several authors (Fagan and Pabon 1990). A 1996 study by the American Council on Education (1997) found that among the major ethnic groups, Hispanics had the lowest high school completion rates (53.0%). The U.S. Bureau of the Census (1993) found the dropout rate among Hispanic youth (27.5%) to be more than twice as high as the rate for African American youth (13.6%) and more than three times as high as the rate for white youth (7.9%). The effect of poverty is quite apparent when stratifying Hispanic youth, ages 16–24, by low family income—the dropout rate increases to nearly one-half (44.7%) of all Hispanic youth (U.S. Bureau of the Census 1995). Studies (Kolstad and Kaufman 1989) indicated that Hispanic dropouts were less likely than others to return to school. Kolstad and Kaufman's study reported that only 39% of the Hispanics had returned to school or enrolled in general equivalency diploma classes compared with 51% of the African Americans and 54% of the whites. These trends are particularly disheartening because dropouts are more difficult to reach with school-based rehabilitative efforts. They are at considerably higher risk for progressing to chronic substance use and developing serious drug-related problems (Chavez 1993). It is also essential to recognize that drug use itself is frequently a contributing factor in the downward spiral that may lead to the Hispanic student leaving the educational system.

The aggressive marketing by the alcohol and tobacco industry to promote the purchase of their products especially targets Hispanics because the youthfulness and growth of the Hispanic population make it a very profitable market ("Beer Markets" 1989). The corporate marketing strategies are aimed at legitimizing and encouraging alcohol and tobacco use among the Hispanic population without regard for the often-disastrous health consequences. Because several studies (Ruiz and Langrod 1997) have found that Hispanic youth are significantly less informed about the ill effects of alcohol, tobacco, and other drugs than are their white counterparts, it is all the more disconcerting that Hispanics are expressly targeted. This deficient knowledge base among Hispanics translates to a decrease in the perceived risk of using alcohol and tobacco, which correlates with more extensive use of these substances. Researchers (McMahon and Taylor 1990) have consistently noted the ubiquitous and disproportionately higher number of alcohol retail outlets and tobacco and alcohol billboards permeating predominantly low-income Hispanic and African American communities. In addition to the increased availability of alcohol and tobacco, the availability of illicit drugs such as crack cocaine and marijuana in impoverished Hispanic communities has expanded since the late 1980s (Castro 1994). The recent resurgence of heroin use among Hispanics is in large measure the result of its expanded presence in Hispanic communities (Castro 1994).

In concluding this discussion of the factors relevant to substance abuse among Hispanics, it should be noted that federal, state, and local governments spend $30 billion annually in the United States on illicit drug control (D. G. Lewis, Director, Brown University Center for Alcohol and Addiction Studies, statement at press conference following meeting of Physician Leadership on National Drug Policy, July 9, 1997). About three-fourths of these expenditures are funneled into the criminal justice system in an ineffectual strategy to curtail drug use (D. G. Lewis, Director, Brown University Center for Alcohol and Addiction Studies, statement at press conference following meeting of Physician Leadership on National Drug Policy, July 9, 1997). The unfortunate result has been to obfuscate society's recognition of the need to prioritize prevention, treatment, and rehabilitation. The large diversion of Hispanics into the criminal justice system for minor drug offenses has engendered in many of them a strong sense of anger, victimization, and alienation from mainstream society. This is commonly a factor in their continuing to use drugs after being released from correctional facilities.

CULTURAL ISSUES IN
SUBSTANCE ABUSE TREATMENT

The literature on the subject of substance abuse among Hispanic Americans suggests that cultural factors play a prominent role in initiating and maintaining drug use (Kail 1993). A distinctive characteristic of Hispanic culture is the importance of the family. *Familismo* is the trait that describes the family as the center of social support and characterizes it as a source of solidarity, cohesiveness, and emotional closeness (Sanchez Mayers and Kail 1993). Family members are imbued with a strong sense of responsibility to one another. It is relevant to mention that although a strength of the Hispanic person is the importance of the family unit, this cultural trait also may discourage help seeking in the Hispanic drug user. Consequently, preventive and treatment efforts must include the family, whenever possible, but especially when adolescents are identified as substance abusers.

One of the most extensively studied of all cultural constructs of Hispanics is acculturation, which refers to the social and psychological process whereby immigrants and their offspring adopt the values, attitudes, and behaviors of the host culture. The relation of acculturation to substance abuse among Hispanics has at times been unclear and dependent on the theoretical perspective used by researchers to define acculturation. Most research on acculturation (Garza and Gallegos 1995) has used simplistic, one-dimensional models that do not address the constellation of variables that affect the Hispanic individual in adjusting to United States society. The weight of the literature does suggest that higher levels of acculturation to United States society, as reflected by English language use, is associated with higher levels of drug use (Kail 1993). It has been postulated that Hispanic youth who are more acculturated than their parents may bond less to them, resulting in a less cohesive family unit. Because research (De La Rosa 1988) has suggested that the family plays a more important role as a social support network for Hispanics than it does for either whites or African Americans, the consequences of a disruption in these ties can be more severe for Hispanic youth. The correlation between alcohol intake and acculturation among Hispanics is probably the least ambiguous of the various drug associations studied (Caetano 1987). The bulk of the literature links increased drinking frequency with increased acculturation (Caetano 1987). Studies of Hispanic men have found variable degrees of consistency with this association, depending on which particular subgroup was examined and how acculturation was measured (Caetano 1987). The association between acculturation and drinking is more robust among Hispanic women (Caetano 1987). The frequency and quantity of alcohol ingestion is greater,

especially among employed and highly acculturated Hispanic women (Caetano 1987). For Hispanics in general, those highly acculturated but least
educated are most likely to report the greatest drug use (Kail 1993). The realities of discrimination, entrapment in poverty, and disillusionment with not
achieving upward socioeconomic mobility serve to alienate Hispanics from
mainstream United States society. This may galvanize them to use drugs, regardless of their level of acculturation.

The trait of fatalism is one that has been well described in the Hispanic
population (Soriano 1994). It is, nonetheless, difficult to ascribe the construct
of fatalism to Hispanics entirely as a cultural trait because of the disproportionate level of socioeconomic hardship faced by Hispanics. Simply being a
minority and living under oppressive conditions with limited access to the opportunity structure in the United States may engender feelings of hopelessness and contribute to a fatalistic attitude. Some scholars postulated that
emphasizing the fatalism to Hispanics, with its implied sense of passivity and
resignation, has played a role in advancing certain pejorative views of Hispanics (Soriano 1994). A particularly draconian misconception among some clinicians is that Hispanics are not as motivated as other groups to seek treatment
(Soriano 1994). This false belief in poor motivation often serves as a conve-
nient excuse for drug treatment programs to not review and modify policies
and practices to facilitate the Hispanic patient's seeking and remaining in
treatment. A careful analysis of several of these "unmotivated" cases has very
often indicated that the Hispanic patient was not responsive to a specific treatment, but when matched to a more appropriate intervention, she or he showed
considerably greater engagement and retention in treatment.

The ethnocultural value that demarcates gender roles in Hispanic men is
known as *machismo*. A fairly acceptable definition of *machismo* is that it is a set
of traits expected of the Hispanic male, wherein he, as the provider, has a duty
to and responsibility for the welfare of his family. Selected aspects of the construct of *machismo* are particularly relevant in the treatment of substance
abuse in Hispanics and have important implications for the prevention of drug
abuse. *Machismo* may contribute significantly to the pervasiveness of substance abuse in the Hispanic community by fostering considerable denial in
the Hispanic drug abuser. The Hispanic male often avoids presenting for substance abuse treatment because it is perceived as an admission of weakness or
poor coping ability and may result in considerable shame and humiliation. Of
course, the degree to which the Hispanic male relates to *machismo* varies considerably. Another behavior that may be considerably influenced by *machismo*
is the desire to drink alcohol in large quantities without showing intoxication
or loss of self-control. A growing body of evidence (Schuckit 1994) indicates

that a low level of response or reduced sensitivity to alcohol, especially among the sons of alcoholic patients, is a potent predictor of future alcoholism. In light of these research findings, it is advisable that clinicians educate their Hispanic patients about the increased risk of developing alcohol dependency if they have a family history of alcoholism or an enhanced ability to "hold their liquor." Because drinking alcohol has such deeply ingrained associations with *machismo,* the warning that outdrinking others should not be viewed as a prized trait must be vigorously repeated.

Clinicians must be sensitive to the possibility that certain treatment options may not always be appropriate if a particular Hispanic patient shows a strong identification with the construct of *machismo.* A common example of this is the ambivalence of some Hispanics to embrace the 12 steps of Alcoholics Anonymous (AA). The notion of admitting to being powerless over alcohol, as is stated in step 1 of the AA creed, may strike a painful chord in the Hispanic who much of his or her life may have felt the powerlessness and diminished sense of self-worth that frequently stems from being a minority in the United States. In this individual, the religious appeal of a "higher power" in AA may not be enough to compensate for feeling disempowered. He or she may opt for a program with a different focus, such as Rational Recovery (Trimpey 1992), that stresses a more cognitive approach to maintaining sobriety. For thousands of other Hispanics, however, AA and the other 12-step programs have been a valuable resource and, when appropriate, should be considered as part of any treatment plan. Clinicians should attempt to determine whether a particular self-help group is for Spanish-speaking persons and/or sensitive to the Hispanic person's culture before referring the patient.

Hispanics generally ascribe considerable importance to their sense of dignity and honor. Clinicians should be highly sensitive to comments or actions that may transgress the substance abuser's sense of dignity, which is already probably tarnished from living in a society that holds drug users in contempt. The failure of substance abuse programs to retain Hispanics is often a result of the confrontational style sometimes used by staff, which may be viewed by Hispanic patients as an affront to their dignity. The clinician may find it useful to explain the rationale for certain procedures to patients beforehand to avoid impugning their character, especially with the thorny issue of compulsory urine drug testing. It is beneficial to explain to the patient that urine testing is a method of gauging the effectiveness of substance abuse treatment and that it is not performed with the express purpose of "catching the patient in a lie." The clinician can help the patient understand that the nature of an addictive illness is such that it may preclude the patient's being truthful on certain occasions, regardless of the patient's well-intentioned efforts or inherently honest character.

Religion or a sense of spirituality is often a major influence in the lives of Hispanics and is a source of comfort in times of stress. In those persons who have a high degree of religious motivation, this approach has produced results (Muffler et al. 1992) that are comparable to those of other traditional forms of treatment. For those Hispanics who have dissolved ties with their families and friends as a consequence of their drug use, a religious faith can function as a support system and provide a much-needed sense of fellowship. One of the best examples is the work of Reverend Cecil Williams (Williams and Laird 1992), pastor of Glide Memorial Church in San Francisco, California, who has successfully used a spiritual approach termed *a spirituality of recovery* to empower members of his congregation to overcome addictions. His theology of recovery may have special appeal to the Hispanic substance abuser living in privation and struggling with an inauspicious sense of the future. "Recovery simply means opening the door to the possibilities. Life awaits," are the words Williams used to describe the essence of his spiritual approach. Clinicians should certainly not assume, however, that every Hispanic individual will find a religious approach to treatment helpful.

PRINCIPLES OF SUBSTANCE ABUSE TREATMENT

A central doctrine in the drug treatment of Hispanic Americans is the need to match the patient to the most appropriate form of care. Unfortunately, the "one-size-fits-all" approach to substance abuse treatment is still evident in many clinics throughout the United States. These treatment agencies often lack Spanish-speaking, culturally competent staff who understand and are sensitive to the particular cultural characteristics of their patients. Because it is frequently not possible to have a bilingual and bicultural therapist available, the therapist assigned to a Hispanic patient should be at least knowledgeable and understanding of Hispanic cultural values and beliefs. The ability of the therapist to effectively integrate the value systems of the Hispanic individual and of United States society as they relate to the substance abuse problems of the patient is crucial. It is equally vital to be on guard against making assumptions of the patient's needs and potential response to treatment on the basis of blanket cultural generalizations that may not be warranted. Thus, those particular cultural values that apply to the patient's own subgroup and the personal qualities of the patient must be taken into consideration.

One of the best examples of tailoring a particular therapy to a specific Hispanic subgroup has been the work of Szapocznik and Kurtines (1989), who successfully used their strategic structural-systems engagement to treat drug use in Cuban Americans and their families. Szapocznik's approach is culturally sensitive because it strengthens the role of parents in the traditionally hierarchical Hispanic family and because it is well suited to address problems of intergenerational conflict that arise from migration and acculturation (Rio et al. 1990). The functioning extended family is portrayed as a source of strength and a preventer of drug use, whereas the fragmented or dysfunctional family is described as a source of disruption and demoralization that leads to drug use (Rio et al. 1990).

When the Hispanic patient first presents to the treatment provider, it is highly recommended that the issue of confidentiality be explained to the patient's full satisfaction. The objective is to engender as much trust as possible in the clinical setting and promote therapeutic disclosure. Scores of Hispanics may have been exposed to regimes in their countries of origin that involved limited freedoms and considerable surveillance, resulting in their having little trust in institutions. To foster the honest communication of sensitive material, the therapist must be nonjudgmental about the patient's drug use and convey respect, empathy, and a sense of equality at all times. This nonjudgmental approach by the clinician is immensely important because it is often the most influential of all the factors affecting the Hispanic patient's decision to remain in treatment. Many Hispanics are extremely reticent to seek treatment because of the shame society attaches to being a drug user, particularly if they live in areas of the United States where anti-immigrant xenophobia has crossed over into anti-Hispanic sentiment. Research (Delgado and Hume-Delgado 1993) has indicated that Hispanics often ascribe to a nondisease, or moral, model of addiction wherein the drug user is stigmatized and labeled as lacking in moral fortitude or having a "weak character." For these reasons, it is understandable that the Hispanic patient can often be exquisitely sensitive to any indication that the clinician may be passing judgment on his or her drug use.

Because of the additional culturally based stigma experienced by the substance-abusing Hispanic female, and the special treatment needs (e.g., pregnancy) of women, employment of female staff is clearly indicated, whenever possible. Also, at the first meeting with the Hispanic patient, the clinician should inquire about the specific Hispanic subgroup to which the patient belongs. This shows respect for the uniqueness of the patient's culture and enhances rapport. Ultimately, any intervention that improves the alliance between the patient and the clinician is extremely valuable when the highly charged topic of substance abuse is the focus of discussion.

In working with the Hispanic substance abuser, it has been found efficacious to focus on the "here and now" in therapy, based on the assumption that this is more consistent with cultural expectations and with the realities of those Hispanics in deprived socioeconomic circumstances. The clinician may find it helpful to engage the patient in therapy that is pragmatic, catalytic, and problem solving in its orientation. A cognitive-behavioral (Beck et al. 1993) approach, in particular, fulfills many of these characteristics and has proven to be effective when tailored to relapse prevention. The cognitive approach helps to reduce the intensity and frequency of the urges to use drugs by modifying the underlying erroneous thinking and maladaptive beliefs. A particular challenge in therapy is redirecting Hispanic substance abusers into the preventive mode of thinking in relation to their drug use, when many are in the survival mode because of economically disadvantaged situations. Another major challenge for the clinician is to not overemphasize the significance of the disease model of addiction when educating the Hispanic patient about the addiction process. The danger is that the patient may feel predestined to continue with his or her alcohol or drug use, especially if he or she already has a strong degree of fatalism as part of his or belief system. The clinician must inform his or her patient that although he or she may have a predisposition or heightened vulnerability to substance abuse, he or she is certainly not predestined to become addicted to drugs. This therapeutic approach empowers the Hispanic patient to assume a strong measure of responsibility for the drug use and not abdicate the role as an active participant in treatment and recovery.

A point of considerable contention when a Hispanic patient initially presents for an evaluation of substance use is to what extent an actual alcohol or drug problem exists. To accurately answer this question and not risk alienating the patient, the clinician must thoroughly review with the Hispanic individual the criteria for making this determination. Many in the addiction field have realized that clinicians cannot solely rely on measures of quantity and frequency of drug use to diagnose abuse or dependence. Some clinicians may overrely on these measures and neglect other criteria that are more salient in determining whether a substance use problem exists. The clinician should emphasize to Hispanic patients that the sine qua non for a drug use problem is a loss of control that is best demonstrated by the patient's continuing to use of a drug even though using creates significant life problems. The ability of certain Hispanic patients to intermittently curtail or discontinue their drug use, only to eventually start again, also is often erroneously interpreted by the patient as signifying that "there is really not a problem." The clinician must educate the Hispanic patient that this pattern simply represents the chronic, relapsing nature of the addiction process and that it most assuredly indicates that treatment is necessary.

A significant proportion of clinicians treating substance abuse believe that alcohol- and drug-related problems frequently develop because of an individual's attempt to self-medicate a psychiatric condition. However, a careful review of the literature by Schuckit (Brown and Schuckit 1988; Schuckit and Hesselbrock 1994) indicated that about 60%–70% of the people who develop serious alcohol or drug problems do not have a major preexisting psychiatric disorder. Their substance abuse is actually the primary disorder and often leads to the development of secondary psychiatric symptoms. If this appears to be the case after taking a careful history and delineating the temporal sequence of symptoms in a patient, it is helpful to inform the patient that symptoms of depression or anxiety may be temporary and disappear on their own with abstinence. Note, however, that certain psychiatric diagnoses in Hispanics, especially posttraumatic stress disorder, often are associated with a significant degree of self-medication with alcohol and drugs. All patients must therefore be followed up once they achieve abstinence to ensure that their psychiatric symptoms remit. If symptoms remain, a psychiatric assessment is certainly warranted. It is also judicious for the clinician to inquire whether the patient has been given any medications by friends or relatives who may have sought to help relieve the patient's distress by sharing their own supply. This is a very culturally sanctioned practice among many Hispanics but may seriously complicate the patient's substance abuse treatment if the provider is unaware. Many medications that have significant abuse potential, such as diazepam, can be obtained without a prescription in some countries in Latin America and may lead to unsupervised and indiscriminate use in the United States.

As stated earlier in the chapter, Hispanic women may underreport their alcohol use because of the austere cultural proscriptions they face when drinking. Clinicians must stress to all Hispanic female drinkers of childbearing age, whether known to be pregnant or not, that there is no known safe level of alcohol consumption during pregnancy and that they should abstain completely if possible. Some are tragically unaware that although they may deliver apparently healthy babies without physical signs of fetal alcohol syndrome, myriad neuropsychiatric problems are attributable to gestational alcohol intake, such as speech and language delays, learning disabilities, and emotional instability, which sometimes do not become evident until well after birth. It is helpful for clinicians to present balanced points of view to their Hispanic patients when the media sensationalize a particular drug issue. For example, the past media reports of low to moderate alcohol ingestion reducing cholesterol levels usually have failed to emphasize to the public that such benefits are far outweighed by the colossal health problems that can arise from alcohol abuse. In a similar vein, the favorable publicity recently generated for marijuana because of its medically approved uses has caused many Hispanics to perceive it as harmless.

Now is an opportune time to return to a discussion of the catastrophic association of substance abuse and AIDS and the ramifications for clinicians treating these high-risk Hispanics. When substance abuse, especially injection drug use, is added to inadequate access to health care and the often deplorable socioeconomic conditions faced by Hispanics, it is evident why this population has been so severely and disproportionately affected by the AIDS epidemic. Research (National Center for Health Statistics 1989) has consistently shown that Hispanics are the least knowledgeable of all racial/ethnic groups about AIDS, HIV transmission, and methods of prevention, whereas a definite correlation has been found between years of education and the perceived risk of HIV infection. Hispanics are at higher risk than other groups for HIV infection because of increased rates of injection drug use and greater sharing of needles and drug paraphernalia (Friedman et al. 1986). In addition, the natural disdain for needles that may serve as a deterrent in many cultures may be tempered significantly in certain Hispanic populations in which use of needles to administer antibiotics and vitamins to family members is not uncommon (Marín and Marín 1989). Several studies (Stimson et al. 1990) funded by the Centers for Disease Control and Prevention in the United States and others abroad have provided strong evidence that the availability of clean needles in needle-exchange programs reduces the rate of HIV transmission among those who inject drugs and does not increase the rate of injection drug use. It is clear that the ban on many needle-exchange programs and methadone maintenance programs is less the result of a scientific analysis of these interventions and more the result of uninformed officials engaging in vitriolic rhetoric to advance their political agendas. Government officials and politicians remain loath to endorse any AIDS prevention strategy that may be viewed as sanctioning illicit drug use. The often-heard but ill-advised drug enforcement mantra, "We don't want to send the wrong message," is far removed from the reality that needle-exchange programs do not increase the rate of injection drug use and do save lives by reducing HIV transmission. Although these programs are not sufficient by themselves, they are certainly an improvement over other methods of preventing HIV transmission in the drug injecting population. It is crucial that clinicians treating substance abuse in Hispanics realize that needle-exchange programs also may serve as the initial entry point of a patient into a drug treatment program and be a vehicle for disseminating vital information about risk reduction. The need to improve access to treatment was borne out by a National Institute on Drug Abuse study (National Drug and Alcoholism Treatment Unit Survey 1991), which showed that about 45% of Hispanic intravenous drug users have never been in treatment. The consequences of denying needle-exchange and methadone maintenance programs to the exceptionally vulnerable Hispanic population are potentially cataclysmic.

In concluding this discussion of HIV transmission in the Hispanic population, it should not be lost on clinicians that the use of any drugs, regardless of whether injected or not, can result in HIV infection by leading to other high-risk behaviors. When other factors that adversely affect the Hispanic person's immune function, such as poverty, malnutrition, and poor access to health care, are also considered, we can appreciate why Hispanics are such a susceptible population and have an augmented risk of HIV infection.

Clinicians also must have an open mind toward the use of nontraditional treatments that could prove successful in certain cases. One example is the use of acupuncture in treating opiate and cocaine addiction. Acupuncture has gained wide acceptance in Latin America and Europe, but until recently, its use in the United States has been limited to certain large centers. Although there is skepticism about its efficacy because it has been difficult to conduct controlled clinical trials, acupuncture should certainly remain an option for the motivated Hispanic patient. It may prove particularly beneficial in the Hispanic individual who has failed other treatment modalities or has a history of a good response to acupuncture in his or her country of origin.

Clinicians working with recidivistic Hispanic patients must realize how important alcohol or drugs have become in their patients' lives. This can assuage the clinician's frustration when treating a patient prone to relapse and assist that clinician in continuing to work constructively toward his or her patient's recovery.

The following brief case report illustrates some of the more salient issues in treating substance abuse in the Hispanic patient.

> Mr. S, a 37-year-old Mexican American unemployed construction worker, conversant mostly in Spanish, was referred to the Family Treatment Center by his wife for excessive drinking and difficulty in getting along with the other members of the family. According to his wife, Mr. S had become increasingly irritable, argumentative, and depressed and had begun to drink alcohol frequently and in large amounts in the weeks following the loss of his job.
>
> At the outset of therapy, Mr. S was reluctant to discuss the difficulties at home, stating often that "anyone else out of work would also be having a rough time" and that he was entitled to drink to cope with his disappointment. The therapist empathized with the problems Mr. S was facing but was clear in the first meeting that to derive any benefit from therapy, Mr. S would have to refrain from all alcohol use. The therapist acknowledged the challenging nature of this task and stated that he would wholeheartedly support Mr. S in his struggle to achieve abstinence. He impressed on Mr. S that his

problem with alcohol was not a sign of weakness but a disease that he could recover from. The therapist helped Mr. S understand that drinking was exceedingly detrimental to his daily functioning and impeded his effectiveness as the head of the family. This allowed Mr. S to counteract derision from friends, maintain his dignity, and remain invested in treatment.

In the initial sessions, the therapist allowed Mr. S wide latitude and considerable time to describe his expectations of treatment. Following this, a detailed accounting of Mr. S's alcohol use and its effect on his functioning was obtained. Mr. S agreed to pursue additional treatment for his alcohol abuse but vehemently opposed a referral to a Spanish-speaking AA group on the grounds that he was not "religious" and had felt uncomfortable with the AA doctrine that he was "powerless" over alcohol. He stated that his preference was to learn how he could help himself and not feel dependent on others to maintain his sobriety. After further discussion, the therapist believed that a referral to a Spanish-speaking Rational Recovery Systems group might be a better match for Mr. S's belief system.

The therapist then referred Mr. S to a seminar at the treatment center that focused on dealing with unemployment and searching for a new job. Soon after attending the seminar, Mr. S was able to discuss some of his other stressors in therapy. He admitted feeling that he had "let down" his family because he was not able to contribute financially and expressed particular shame after friends joked that his wife, who was a seamstress, was "supporting" him. He also was unable to continue sending money to his mother in Mexico, which had always been a great source of pride for him. After several weeks, Mr. S further confided that having to depend on his three children to translate into Spanish had always caused him to feel weak and "not in charge," exacerbating his sense of helplessness.

As therapy progressed, Mr. S gradually began to view treatment as less stigmatizing and more helpful. This was partially accomplished by the therapist's successfully reducing Mr. S's resistance to admitting that he had lost control of his drinking without impugning his manhood. The therapist guided Mr. S in refocusing on the fact that by seeking assistance and acknowledging his problems, Mr. S was also helping his family to get through this difficult period. The therapist was able to successfully appeal to Mr. S's sense of *machismo* by promoting the reality that by abstaining from alcohol, Mr. S was actually reinforcing his position as the head of the family.

In the later stages of treatment, the therapist was able to help Mr. S challenge some of the distorted cognitions relating to his alcohol abuse, including his grossly exaggerated sense of the number of men who drank alcohol to cope with stress. Mr. S came to realize that several individuals in his neighborhood were experiencing economic hardship but had not resorted to drinking. He was more open to other suggestions for improving his situation, including enrolling in an English as a second language class to increase his English-speaking ability and, thereby, also improve his self-esteem because of a reduced reliance on his children to translate.

Near the termination of his therapy and with Mr. S's consent, the therapist invited Mrs. S to help her better understand the principal issues associated with Mr. S's drinking. The therapist also used the opportunity to educate her about alcoholism and discuss ways that she could support her husband in his sobriety. A few days after this meeting, Mr. S continued his job search and decided to apply for unemployment benefits, which he had previously refused to do because of feeling ashamed.

The above case report illustrates some key points that are useful in understanding specific dynamics in working with substance-abusing Hispanic patients. A major task for the therapist was addressing Mr. S's view that his alcohol use was simply an adaptive response to being unemployed. The key to the therapist's success was eventually leading Mr. S to recognize and deal with his alcohol use as an issue independent of the loss of his job. The therapist was able to advance the process by which Mr. S assumed responsibility for his drinking, which led to his patient experiencing a more sanguine sense of the future. The empathic, nonjudgmental, and comprehensive approach used by the therapist greatly enhanced communication with his patient and led to a satisfactory outcome. This case also shows the tremendous importance ascribed to employment in the Hispanic culture and how the therapist's sensitivity to this issue laid the foundation for a trusting alliance and allowed him to effectively engage the patient in a discussion of his alcohol abuse.

CONCLUSIONS

In this chapter, I have presented some key points about the nature and etiology of substance abuse among Hispanic Americans and have provided some practical guidelines for treating substance abuse in the Hispanic patient. Although Hispanics are a very heterogeneous population and the etiology of drug use is complex and multifactorial, a strong effort has been made to underscore the importance of socioeconomic and cultural conditions in the evolution and persistence of drug use in this vulnerable population. It is in the context of these conditions that clinicians can better comprehend the tremendous toll that substance abuse has taken on Hispanics. The extensive drug abuse documented in significant segments of the Hispanic population, especially among youth, is incompatible with a productive and secure existence and is a source of great torment, anguish, and suffering for the many Hispanics affected.

American society has developed a paradigm of condemnation as its primary method of dealing with substance abuse. United States policymakers resist accepting the incontrovertible evidence that drug problems are a symptom of other problems facing Hispanics, such as poverty, discrimination, undereducation, and unemployment. It is clear that the solution to the drug problem must involve solutions to these other problems. The currently flawed

United States drug policy, based disproportionately on law enforcement and an unsophisticated understanding of relevant socioeconomic variables, has done little to ameliorate the ravages of drug addiction among Hispanics. Specious arguments and polarizing rhetoric must be replaced by a policy predicated on reason and scientific inquiry. Future substance abuse research on the Hispanic American population should focus on what treatment is effective for which specific subgroups and under what conditions. Clinicians must better understand why Hispanics initiate drug use so early in life and why the degree of multiple drug use is so high. Well-controlled treatment outcome studies can best nullify the misinformation contributing to the counterproductive societal mindset that tends to criminalize Hispanics and other substance abusers. To attenuate the plague of Hispanic drug abuse, the federal government must enforce a drug policy that is less punitive and more rehabilitative in scope. We cannot expect to eradicate drugs from beleaguered Hispanic communities with prisons serving as the major repository of our hopes for success. Worthwhile initiatives may include increasing drug treatment in the criminal justice setting and expanding judicial processes to offer more treatment alternatives to incarceration for nonviolent offenders.

Clinicians must advocate for comprehensive, integrated human service programs that emphasize prevention and early intervention and target high-risk Hispanics, especially indigent youth. Treatment programs should orchestrate a partnership with schools, churches, and law enforcement and social welfare agencies to reduce the availability of and demand for alcohol and drugs in the Hispanic community. A public health approach that treats addiction as a chronic illness and uses harm-reduction strategies has considerable merit. Agencies and school-based interventions that are committed to preventing school dropouts are greatly needed. These interventions must be supplemented with programs to reach out-of-school youth, given the pronounced dropout rate among Hispanics. Teaching Hispanic youth about substance abuse earlier in the educational process and before the first drug exposure is the blueprint for effective prevention campaigns. Because education is the principal strategy available to deter thousands of Hispanic youth from starting down the road of addiction, the educational messages must be appropriate, culturally relevant, and delivered by individuals who are sensitive to the needs of Hispanic youth. To have the greatest likelihood of succeeding, these programs should be staffed by bilingual, culturally competent clinicians who can respond flexibly to a wide variety of social, educational, and health needs. As illustrated in the case example, supportive relationships, the availability of a satisfying job, and skills training are key factors in the successful rehabilitation of the Hispanic substance abuser. Treatment providers need to continue to advocate on behalf of patients to guarantee equitable allocation of resources because our society often turns a deaf ear to the plight of the substance abuser.

In conclusion, clinicians must be indefatigable in promoting the belief to Hispanic patients that their substance abuse problems are not insurmountable but possible to overcome with knowledge and active participation in treatment. Through the treatment approaches outlined in this chapter, we can bring dignity and meaning back to the lives of those Hispanic Americans afflicted by the scourge of substance abuse.

REFERENCES

Aguirre-Molina M, Caetano R: Alcohol use and alcohol-related issues, in Latino Health in the US: A Growing Challenge. Edited by Molina CW, Aguirre-Molina M. Washington, DC, American Public Health Association, 1994, pp 400–401

American Council on Education: Minorities in Higher Education: Annual Report. Washington, DC, American Council on Education, 1997

Beck AT, Wright FD, Newman CF: Cognitive Therapy of Substance Abuse. New York, Guilford, 1993

Beer markets vie for black and Hispanic dollars. Pennsylvania Liquor Observer, June 21, 1989

Booth MW, Castro FG, Anglin MD: What do we know about Hispanic substance abuse? A review of the literature, in Drugs in Hispanic Communities. Edited by Glick R, Moore J. New Brunswick, NJ, Rutgers University Press, 1990, pp 21–40

Botvin GJ, Schinke S, Orlandi MA: Drug Abuse Prevention With Multiethnic Youth. Thousand Oaks, CA, Sage, 1995

Brown S, Schuckit MA: Changes in depression among abstinent alcoholics. J Stud Alcohol 49:412–417, 1988

Caetano R: Ethnicity and drinking practices in northern California: a comparison among whites, blacks and Hispanics. Alcohol 19:31–34, 1984

Caetano R: Acculturation and drinking patterns among U.S. Hispanics. British Journal of Addiction 82:789–799, 1987

Caetano R: Alcohol use among Hispanic groups in the United States. Am J Drug Alcohol Abuse 14:293–308, 1988

Castro FG: Drug use and drug-related issues, in Latino Health in the United States: A Growing Challenge. Edited by Molina CW, Aguirre-Molina M. Washington, DC, American Public Health Association, 1994, pp 425–441

Centers for Disease Control and Prevention: Attempted suicide among high school students—United States, 1990. MMWR Morb Mortal Wkly Rep 40:633–635, 1991

Centers for Disease Control and Prevention: National Health Interview Survey, Youth Risk Behavior Survey. Atlanta, GA, Centers for Disease Control and Prevention, 1992

Centers for Disease Control and Prevention: Youth Risk Behavior Surveillance System, 1995. Atlanta, GA, Centers for Disease Control and Prevention, 1995

Centers for Disease Control and Prevention: HIV/AIDS Surveillance Report 8(2):11–13, 1996

Chavez EL: Hispanic dropouts and drug use: a review of the literature and methodological considerations, in National Institute on Drug Abuse: Drug Abuse Among Minority Youth: Methodological Issues and Recent Research Advances (NIDA Res Monogr 130; NIH Publ No 93-3479). Edited by De La Rosa MR, Recio Adrados JL. Washington, DC, U.S. Government Printing Office, 1993, pp 224–232

Chavez EL, Swaim RC: Hispanic substance abuse: problems in epidemiology, in Ethnic and Multicultural Drug Abuse: Perspectives on Current Research. Edited by Trimble JE, Bolek CS, Niemcryk SJ. Binghamton, NY, Harrington Park Press, 1992, pp 211–228

De La Rosa MR: Natural support systems of Hispanics: a key dimension for their well-being. Health Soc Work 15:181–190, 1988

Delgado M, Hume-Delgado D: Chemical dependence, self-help groups, and the Hispanic community, in Hispanic Substance Abuse. Edited by Sanchez Mayers R, Kail BL, Watts TD. Springfield, IL, Charles C Thomas, 1993, pp 145–156

Fagan JA, Pabon E: Contributions of delinquency and substance use to school dropout among inner-city youths. Youth and Society 21(3):306–354, 1990

Felix-Ortiz M, Munoz R, Newcomb MD: The Role of Emotional Distress in Drug Use Among Latino Adolescents. Journal of Child and Adolescent Substance Abuse 3:1–18, 1994

Fernandez-Pol B, Bluestone H, Missouri C, et al: Drinking patterns of inner-city black Americans and Puerto Ricans. J Stud Alcohol 47:156–160, 1986

Friedman S, Des Jarlais D, Sotheran J: AIDS health education for intravenous drug users. Health Education Quarterly 13:383–393, 1986

Garza RT, Gallegos PI: Environmental influences and personal choice: a humanistic perspective on acculturation, in Hispanic Psychology: Critical Issues in Theory and Research. Edited by Padilla AM. Thousand Oaks, CA, Sage, 1995, pp 3–14

Gilbert MJ: Alcohol-related practices, problems and norms among Mexican-Americans: an overview, in Alcohol Use Among US Ethnic Minorities. Rockville, MD, National Institute on Alcohol Abuse and Alcoholism, 1985, pp 115–134

Gold MS: Cocaine (and crack): clinical aspects, in Substance Abuse: A Comprehensive Textbook, 3rd Edition. Edited by Lowinson JH, Ruiz P, Millman RB, et al. Baltimore, MD, Williams & Wilkins, 1992, pp 205–218

Greig A: The war on drugs: who says it's about winning or losing? Harm Reduction Communication, Spring, No. 2, 1996, pp 7–8

Huba GJ, Wingard JA, Bentler PM: Intentions to use drugs among adolescents: a longitudinal analysis. Int J Addict 16:331–339, 1981

Johnston LD, O'Malley PM, Bachman JG (eds): Drug Use Among American High School Seniors, College Students and Young Adults, 1975–1990, Vols 1 and 2 (NIDA DHHS Publ No 91-1813). Washington, DC, U.S. Government Printing Office, 1991

Kail BL: Patterns and predictors of drug abuse within the Chicano community, in Hispanic Substance Abuse. Edited by Sanchez Mayers R, Kail BL, Watts TD. Springfield, IL, Charles C Thomas, 1993, pp 19–36

Kandel D, Yamaguchi K: From beer to crack: developmental patterns in drug involvement. Am J Public Health 83:851–855, 1993

Kolstad AJ, Kaufman P: Dropouts who complete high school with a diploma or GED. Paper presented at the American Educational Research Association, San Francisco, CA, May 1989

Maddahian E, Newcomb MD, Bentler PM: Single and multiple patterns of adolescent substance abuse: longitudinal comparisons of four ethnic groups. J Drug Educ 15:311–326, 1985

Marín BV, Marín G: Information About Human Immunodeficiency Virus in Hispanics in San Francisco (Technical Report 4). San Francisco, University of California, Center for AIDS Prevention Studies, 1989

Mata A, Rodriguez-Andrew S: Inhalant abuse in a small rural south Texas community: a social epidemiological overview, in Epidemiology of Inhalant Abuse: An Update (NIDA Res Monogr 85). Edited by Crider RA, Rouse BA. Washington, DC, U.S. Government Printing Office, 1988, pp 172–203

McMahon E, Taylor P: Citizens Action Handbook on Alcohol and Tobacco Billboards Advertising. Washington, DC, Center for Science in the Public Interest, 1990

Mensch BS, Kandel DB: Underreporting of substance use in a national longitudinal youth cohort. Public Opinion Quarterly 52:100–124, 1988

Muffler J, Langrod JG, Larson D: "There is a balm in Gilead": religion and substance abuse treatment, in Substance Abuse: A Comprehensive Textbook, 3rd Edition. Edited by Lowinson JH, Ruiz P, Millman RB, et al. Baltimore, MD, Williams & Wilkins, 1992, pp 584–594

National Center for Health Statistics: AIDS Knowledge and Attitudes of Hispanic Americans: Provisional Data From the National Health Interview Survey (DHHS Publ No 89-1250, Adv Data No 166). Hyattsville, MD, National Center for Health Statistics, U.S. Public Health Service, 1989

National Center for Health Statistics. Vital Statistics of the US, 1987, Vol 2: Mortality, Part A (DHHS Publ No 90-1101). Washington, DC, U.S. Public Health Service, 1990

National Drug and Alcoholism Treatment Unit Survey: 1989 Final Report, National Institute on Drug Abuse, AIDS Demonstration Research National Database, May 1991

National Institute on Drug Abuse: National Survey Results on Drug Use From the Monitoring the Future Study, 1975–1993 (NIH Publ No. 94-3809). Washington, DC, U.S. Government Printing Office, 1994

National Institute on Drug Abuse: Drug Use Among Racial/Ethnic Minorities (NIH Publ No 95-3888). Rockville, MD, Division of Epidemiology and Prevention Research, National Institute on Drug Abuse, 1995, pp 13–92

Oetting ER, Beauvais F: Adolescent drug use: findings of national and local surveys. J Clin Consult Psychol 58:385–394, 1990

Porter K, Shapiro I, Barancik S: Shortchanged: Recent Developments in Hispanic Poverty, Income and Employment. Washington, DC, Center on Budget and Policy Priorities, November 1988

Rio A, Santisteban DA, Szapocznik J: Treatment approaches for Hispanic drug-abusing adolescents, in Drugs in Hispanic Communities. Edited by Glick R, Moore J. New Brunswick, NJ, Rutgers University Press, 1990, pp 203–229

Rouse B: Substance abuse in Mexican Americans, in Mental Health Issues of the Mexican Origin Population in Texas: Mental Health Issues of the Mexican Origin Population in Texas: Proceedings of the Fifth Robert L. Sutherland Seminar. Edited by Rodriguez R, Coleman MT. San Antonio, TX, Austin Hogg Foundation for Mental Health, University of Texas, 1986

Ruiz P, Langrod JG: Hispanic Americans, in Substance Abuse: A Comprehensive Textbook, 3rd Edition. Edited by Lowinson JH, Ruiz P, Millman RB, et al. Baltimore, MD, Williams & Wilkins, 1997, pp 705–711

Sanchez Mayers R, Kail BL: Hispanic substance abuse: an overview, in Hispanic Substance Abuse. Edited by Sanchez Mayers R, Kail BL, Watts TD. Springfield, IL, Charles C Thomas, 1993, pp 5–16

Schneider Institute for Health Policy, Brandeis University: Substance Abuse: The Nation's Number One Health Problem. Princeton, NJ, Robert Wood Johnson Foundation, 1993, pp 8–17

Schuckit MA: Low level of response to alcohol as a predictor of future alcoholism. Am J Psychiatry 151:184–189, 1994

Schuckit MA, Hesselbrock V: Alcohol dependence and anxiety disorders: what is the relationship? Am J Psychiatry 151:1723–1734, 1994

Soriano FI: The Latino perspective: a sociocultural portrait, in Managing Multiculturalism in Substance Abuse Services. Edited by Gordon JU. Thousand Oaks, CA, Sage, 1994, pp 117–144

Stimson GV, Dolan K, Donoghue M: The future of UK syringe exchange. International Journal of Drug Policy 2(2):14–17, 1990

Substance Abuse and Mental Health Services Administration: National Household Survey on Drug Abuse, 1993 (DHHS Publ No 94-3017). Washington, DC, U.S. Government Printing Office, 1994

Substance Abuse and Mental Health Services Administration: Data from the Drug Abuse Warning Network (DAWN) 1994 data file. Rockville, MD, Substance Abuse and Mental Health Services Administration, 1994

Sue DW, Sue D: Counseling Hispanic Americans, in Counseling the Culturally Different: Theory and Practice, 2nd Edition. Edited by Sue DW, Sue D. New York, Wiley, 1990, pp 227–242

Szapocznik J, Kurtines WM: Breakthroughs in Family Therapy With Drug-Abusing and Problem Youth. New York, Springer, 1989, pp 3–76

Trimpey J: The Small Book: A Revolutionary Alternative for Overcoming Alcohol and Drug Dependence. New York, Dell, 1992, pp 1–29, 89–105

U.S. Bureau of the Census: Population projections of the U.S. by age, sex, race, and Hispanic origin: 1992 to 2050. Current Population Reports, Series P25-1092. Washington, DC, U.S. Government Printing Office, 1992

U.S. Bureau of the Census: Poverty in the United States: 1992. Current Population Reports, Series P-60, No 185. Washington, DC, U.S. Government Printing Office, 1993

U.S. Bureau of the Census: Current Population Survey, March 1995

U.S. Department of Health and Human Services, Public Health Service, Substance Abuse and Mental Health Services Administration, Drug Abuse Warning Network (DAWN): Annual Medical Examiner Data, 1993

Williams C, Laird R: No Hiding Place: Empowerment and Recovery for Our Troubled Communities. San Francisco, CA, Harper, 1992, pp 15–100

Index

Page numbers printed in *boldface* type refer to tables or figures.